NURSING WITHOUT
BORDERS

VALUES • WISDOM • SUCCESS MARKERS

NURSING WITHOUT BORDERS

Values • Wisdom • Success Markers

Sharon M. Weinstein, MS, RN, CRNI, FAAN
Ann Marie T. Brooks, RN, DNSc, MBA, FAAN, FACHE, FNAP

Sigma Theta Tau International
Honor Society of Nursing®

SIGMA THETA TAU INTERNATIONAL

Editor-in-Chief: Jeff Burnham
Acquisitions Editor: Cynthia Saver, RN, MS
Development Editor: Carla Hall
Copy Editor: Kevin Kent
Editorial Team: Melody Jones, Jane Palmer

Cover Design by: Rebecca Harmon
Interior Design and Page Composition by: Rebecca Harmon

Printed in the United States of America
Printing and Binding by Printing Partners, Indianapolis, Indiana, USA

Sigma Theta Tau International
550 West North Street
Indianapolis, IN 46202

Visit our Web site at **www.nursingsociety.org** and go to the "Publications" link for more information about our books or other publications.

ISBN-10: 1-930538-70-7
ISBN-13: 978-1-930538-70-2

Library of Congress Cataloging-in-Publication Data

Nursing without borders : values, wisdom, success markers / [edited by] Sharon M. Weinstein, Ann Marie T. Brooks.

    p. ; cm.

Includes bibliographical references and index.

    ISBN-13: 978-1-930538-70-2

    ISBN-10: 1-930538-70-7

1. Transcultural nursing. 2. Nursing—International cooperation. I. Weinstein, Sharon. II. Brooks, Ann Marie T., 1947- III. Sigma Theta Tau International.

    [DNLM: 1. Transcultural Nursing. 2. International Cooperation. 3. Nursing Care. WY 107 N9745 2007]

RT86.54.N87 2007

362.17′3—dc22   2007039998

07   08   09   10   11   /   5   4   3   2   1

Photography

The exceptional photography of Barry Kinsella inspired the cover design for *Nursing Without Borders: Values, Wisdom, Success Stories*. He documented Ms. Weinstein's early trips to Russia and beyond. His photographic artwork has documented the lives of people around the world. Barry has been particularly drawn to Eastern European peoples—with a strong focus on the independent states of the former Soviet Union. For his ongoing assignment on behalf of the American International Health Alliance (AIHA) and Premier, Inc., he has created a photographic tribute to hospitals across the United States and their counterparts in countries that were formerly communist. His most recent photographic journeys were to China and Mongolia. Barry's photographs can be viewed at **www.kinsellaphoto.com**.

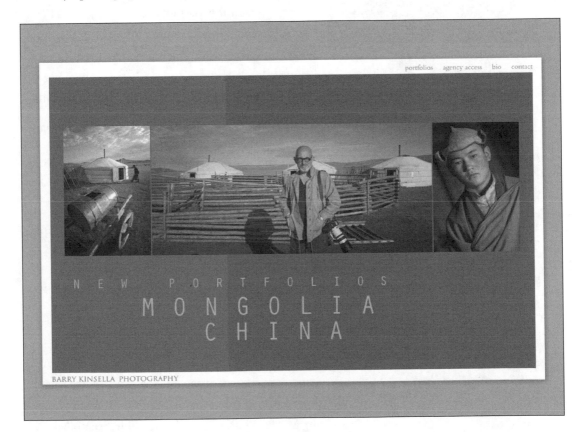

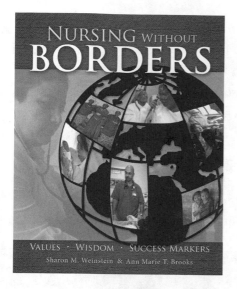

FRONT COVER

Clockwise from top: (1) Sister Anna Mighulo of Kenya; permission to use granted by Marquette University. (2) Central Asian nurse with young patient; © Barry Kinsella (**www.kinsellaphoto.com**). (3) Two Indian Qeqchi girls in their village in Carchá, Guatemala; permission to use granted by Heriberto Herrera, El Salvador (**http://www.sxc. hu/browse.phtml?f=view&id=782525**). (4) Rauf Khalid; photo by Michelle Lilly, Sigma Theta Tau International. (5) Russian nurse with infant; © Barry Kinsella (**www.kinsellaphoto.com**). (6) Background image and first image on left on back cover: Russian nurse with young patient; © Barry Kinsella (**www.kinsellaphoto.com**). (7) Masai men; permission to use granted by Jonathan Hillis (**http://www.sxc.hu/browse.phtml?f=view&id=863 582**).

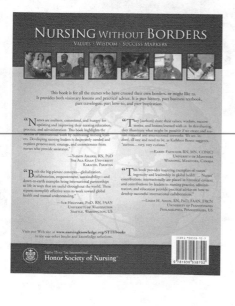

BACK COVER

Left to right: (1) Russian nurse with young patient; © Barry Kinsella (**www.kinsellaphoto.com**). (2) Masai men; permission to use granted by Jonathan Hillis (**http://www.sxc.hu/browse. phtml?f=view&id=863582**). (3) Two Indian Qeqchi girls in their village in Carchá, Guatemala; permission to use granted by Heriberto Herrera, El Salvador (**http://www.sxc.hu/browse. phtml?f=view&id=782525**). (4) Armenian student nurses at Erebouni School of Nursing; © Barry Kinsella (**www.kinsellaphoto.com**). (5) Rauf Khalid; photo by Michelle Lilly, Sigma Theta Tau International. (6) Sister Anna Mighulo of Kenya; permission to use granted by Marquette University.

DEDICATION

Nursing Without Borders: Values, Wisdom, Success Markers is dedicated to nurses worldwide who have mastered the fine art of partnering through collaboration, practice, and education.

We thank Barry Kinsella, the accomplished and internationally recognized photographer who documented our international work. His work is a part of our respective personal collections.

And, we acknowledge the support of our families and friends. International travel and collaboration are challenging. While the demands of international work take time away from home, the opportunity also enriches the lives of those we love.

Publisher's Note: 100% of the author royalties from sales of this book will benefit the Global Education Development Institute (GEDI). For information about GEDI, visit the institute's Web site at **http://www.gedinfp.com/**.

ACKNOWLEDGMENTS

Global nursing impacts health-care delivery in every corner of the world and requires interventions from all sectors of society. *Nursing Without Borders: Values, Wisdom, Success Markers* offers a global perspective on education, process, and practice initiatives. It provides a forum for recognized nurse leaders and activists to share their stories and successes in defining nursing's past, present, and future. Success as a global leader requires a global mind-set, an appreciation of humanities and culture, a sensitivity to diverse human capital, a sense of shared leadership, and accountability.

The international nursing leaders contributing to this text are role models whose stories must be shared. We recognize their accomplishments and goals; we acknowledge their developments and successes; and we thank them for challenging the process, inspiring a shared vision, enabling others to act, and modeling the way for us to go. May they continue to build strategic partnerships in nursing—relationships that will evolve, last a lifetime, and ensure the continued growth of our profession.

With this book, here and now, we invite you to begin the journey to *Nursing Without Borders*.

SHARON M. WEINSTEIN, MS, RN, CRNI, FAAN
ANN MARIE T. BROOKS, RN, DNSc, MBA, FAAN, FACHE, FNAP

ABOUT THE AUTHORS

SHARON M. WEINSTEIN, MS, RN, CRNI, FAAN, is president and founder of the Global Education Development Institute. She facilitated the induction of more than 60 nursing leaders as international members of the Honor Society of Nursing, Sigma Theta Tau International and collaborated with the honor society on the creation of a teaching module for Eastern European nurses called "Leaders for a Scholarly Profession." The author of five books and more than 150 peer-reviewed publications, Weinstein has led international nursing initiatives worldwide for Premier, Inc. as director of international affairs and for the American International Health Alliance as director of nursing partnership programs for the New Independent States of the former Soviet Union and Central and Eastern European countries. She earned a master's degree in health management and gerontology from North Texas State University, a certificate in health administration from Trinity University, a bachelor's degree in nursing and behavioral science from Wilmington College, and a diploma from Pennsylvania Hospital School of Nursing. She is a graduate of the Kellogg Executive Management Program and a member of the American Academy of Nursing's Expert Panel on Global Nursing and Health.

ANN MARIE T. BROOKS, RN, DNSc, MBA, FAAN, FACHE, FNAP, is a nurse executive with extensive leadership and consultation experience in the United States and abroad and is the director of the Vanderbilt-Botswana Project. She is past president of both the American Organization of Nurse Executives (AONE) and the American Psychiatric Nurses Association. She is immediate past dean at The Catholic University of America's School of Nursing. Dr. Brooks is a team leader/mentor for the American Nurse Credentialing Center's Magnet Recognition Program and secretary-treasurer of the Global Education Development Institute. She holds a BSN, MSN, and DNSc from The Catholic University of America and an MBA from Loyola College.

CONTRIBUTING AUTHORS

MARY ALEXANDER

Mary Alexander, RN, CRNI, MA, CAE, is chief executive officer (CEO) of the Infusion Nurses Society (INS) and the Infusion Nurses Certification Corporation (INCC). As CEO, she also serves as the editor of the *Journal of Infusion Nursing*. She recently completed a term of office as president of the American Board of Nursing Specialties. She is a director of the Global Education Institute Board.

JENNIFER ANDREWS

Jennifer Andrews, RN, ADON, is assistant director of nursing, Division of Surgery, at Princess Alexandra Hospital Health Service District in Brisbane, Queensland, Australia, which has achieved Magnet recognition. Her clinical background and experience in leadership roles have provided her with the platform to facilitate and guide clinical practice in the surgical units. She is a frequent presenter at professional society meetings. A graduate of the Princess Alexandra Hospital School of Nursing, she completed specialty training in midwifery and child health.

CLAUDIA BARTZ

Claudia Bartz, PhD, RN, FAAN, is coordinator of International Classification for Nursing Practice and clinical associate professor at the University of Wisconsin-Milwaukee School of Nursing. She retired as a colonel from the United States Army Nurse Corps in 1999 with 30 years of service, having served domestically and internationally.

DEVA-MARIE BECK

Deva-Marie Beck, PhD, RN, is international co-director of the Nightingale Initiative for Global Health. She is a nursing scholar, clinician, health educator, and world ambassador for human health and well-being. She has networked for nursing and transdisciplinary health promotion issues in the United States, Canada, Great Britain, Switzerland, Scandinavia, and Turkey. She has practiced in a wide variety of home-care and critical-care clinical settings in many parts of the world during her more than 30 years of clinical nursing experience.

MARJORIE BEYERS

Marjorie Beyers, EdD, RN, FAAN, is a nursing consultant with a wealth of nurse executive and education experience. She has been actively involved with the Honor Society of Nursing, Sigma Theta Tau International, helping to develop future scenarios, chairing the Finance Committee, and drafting the ARISTA 1 report. She is the former executive director of the American Organization of Nurse Executives (AONE) and system chief nursing officer of Mercy Health Care. Dr. Beyers is a well-known author and international speaker.

KATHLEEN A. BOWER

Kathleen A. Bower, DNSc, RN, FAAN, is principal and co-owner of The Center for Case Management, Inc. She was a member of the team that created clinical paths and provider-based case management at New England Medical Center in 1985. She holds a Bachelor of Science in Nursing from Georgetown University, a Master of Science in Nursing from Boston College, and a doctoral degree in nursing from Boston University.

MARIA HELENA LARCHER CALIRI

Maria Helena Larcher Caliri, RN, PhD, completed postgraduate work at the University of São Paulo, Ribeirão Preto College of Nursing, Brazil, which is a World Health Organization Collaborating Centre for Nursing Research Development. She is currently an associate professor and a researcher.

RITA M. CARTY

Rita M. Carty, PhD, RN, FAAN, is professor and dean emerita of George Mason University, Fairfax, Virginia, USA. Dr. Carty is president emerita of the American Association of Colleges of Nursing and holds the 2002 Sister Bernadette Armiger award. Dr. Carty served as head of George Mason University's College of Nursing and Health Science World Health Organization Collaborating Centre from 1990 to 2006.

AMY COENEN

Amy Coenen, PhD, RN, FAAN, is an associate professor at the University of Wisconsin-Milwaukee College of Nursing. Her research has focused on the nursing minimum data set and terminology standards for the electronic health record. She serves as director of the International Classification for Nursing Practice Programme for the International Council of Nurses. She also serves as a member of the Steering Committee for the International Standards Organization's proposal for a reference terminology model for nursing.

CLARITA D. CURATO

Clarita D. Curato, RN, MAN, EdD, is dean and chief academic officer at De Los Santos – STI College of Healthcare Professions in Quezon City, Philippines.

LEAH CURTIN

Leah Curtin, RN, MS, MA, FAAN, is a clinical professor of nursing at the University of Cincinnati College of Nursing and Health and was editor-in-chief of *Nursing Management* for 20 years. She is director of Cross Country Education's Nurse Manager Boot Camp. She was awarded an honorary doctorate from State University of New York in 1990 for the impact she has had on development of nursing and health care in the United States. In 2002, The Medical College of Ohio awarded her a second honorary doctorate for humanitarian services. She is a prolific writer and popular speaker on a diversity of nursing issues.

ANNE J. DAVIS

Anne J. Davis, RN, PhD, DSc(hon), FAAN, is professor emerita of the University of California, San Francisco and Nagano College of Nursing, Japan. For 45 years, she has worked on numerous international projects. She received the first American Nurses Association Human Rights Award and has been bestowed lifetime honorary professorships at Beijing Medical University and Sun Yat-Sen University in China. She has published more than 200 articles and six books, two of which are in Japanese. At 75 years of age, she remains professionally active by writing and working on short-term international assignments.

RACHEL DIFAZIO

Rachel DiFazio, RN, MS, CPNP, is a pediatric nurse practitioner at Children's Hospital, Boston. She has worked collaboratively with Russian nurses on multiple projects, articles, and educational exchanges and has been the co-coordinator of the US-Russian Nursing Conference Cruise since 2003.

BARBARA M. DOSSEY

Barbara M. Dossey, PhD, RN, AHN-BC, FAAN, is director of Holistic Nursing Consultants and international co-director of the Nightingale Initiative for Global Health. She is a frequent contributor to the nursing literature. Her latest book, *Florence Nightingale: Mystic, Visionary, Healer,* focuses on the philosophical and practical impact of Florence Nightingale's life and work on modern nursing and humankind.

MARIE J. DRIEVER

Marie J. Driever, PhD, RN, is director of professional practice and development, Group Health Cooperative, in Seattle, Washington, USA. She is a clinical nurse researcher whose interest in Russia began with participation in the first US-Russian Nursing Conference Cruise in 1997. Since 2000, Dr. Driever has co-coordinated these conference cruises. The relationships developed from this work have led to her being a member of faculty teams offering conferences on care of the elderly, health care ethics, and nursing research to Russian nurses.

MAJEDA MOHAMMED EL-BANNA

Majeda Mohammed El-Banna, PhD, RN, is associate professor and dean of faculty for nursing at Al-Zaytoonah Private University of Jordan in Amman, Jordan. Her clinical expertise is in adult health nursing, and her academic research is with bone marrow transplant patients and their families, as well as the common symptoms and side effects of bone marrow transplantation. Her BSN and MSN are from the University of Jordan. Her PhD is from the University of Nebraska Medical Center College of Nursing.

CARME ESPINOSA I. FESNEDO

Carme Espinosa I. Fesnedo, RN, BSN, MSc, is with the Universitat d'Andorra and a partici-pant in the Outcome Present State Test (OPT) initiative. A member of the board of directors of Asociación Española de Nomenclatura Taxonomía y Diagnósticos de Enfermería, she is actively involved with the taxonomy, education, and publications committees of NANDA-Internation-al. She is a member of the faculty at the University of Andorra School of Nursing.

ELLEN FINEOUT-OVERHOLT

Ellen Fineout-Overholt, PhD, RN, FNAP, is associate professor of clinical nursing and direc-tor of the Center for the Advancement of Evidence-Based Practice at Arizona State University, Phoenix, Arizona, USA. She received her doctoral degree from the University of Rochester School of Nursing; a master's in nursing from the University of Alabama, Birmingham; and a bachelor's degree in nursing from the University of Texas Medical Branch, Galveston, Texas. She is a frequent contributor to the nursing literature on evidence-based practice.

ANITA FINKELMAN

Anita Finkelman, MSN, RN, is adjunct faculty at the University of Oklahoma School of Nurs-ing. She is president and founder of Resources for Excellence, a consulting firm, and author of several texts addressing leadership, management, and psychiatric nursing.

JOYCE J. FITZPATRICK

Joyce J. Fitzpatrick, PhD, RN, FAAN, is Elizabeth Brooks Ford Professor of Nursing, Frances Payne Bolton School of Nursing at Case Western Reserve University, Cleveland, Ohio, USA, and is editor of *Archives of Psychiatric Nursing*. She received her BSN from Georgetown Univer-sity, an MS in psychiatric-mental health nursing from Ohio State University, a PhD in nursing education from New York University, and an MBA from Case Western Reserve University. She is a renowned researcher, author, and speaker.

JEANNE M. FLOYD

Jeanne M. Floyd, PhD, RN, CAE, FAAN, is executive director of the American Nurses Cre-dentialing Center (ANCC). Before taking over this position at ANCC, Dr. Floyd served as director of strategic development for the Honor Society of Nursing, Sigma Theta Tau Interna-tional. Dr. Floyd earned her PhD from Pennsylvania State University, her MS from the University of Maryland School of Nursing, and her BSN from the College of Notre Dame School of Nursing in Baltimore, Maryland, USA. She also holds a BA from the University of San Francisco Department of Sociology and Social Welfare and a diploma from the Truesdale Hospital School of Nursing in Fall River, Massachusetts, USA.

MARIANNE E. HESS

Marianne E. Hess, BSN, RN, CCRN, is hospital education coordinator of critical care at George Washington University Hospital in Washington, DC, USA. Her international nursing experiences took her from Armenia to Russia. She is a director of the Global Education Development Institute.

MA. KATHERINE O. JIONGCO

Ma. Katherine O. Jiongco, RN, BSN, is staffing services manager with GROW, Inc. based in Makati City, Philippines.

REVEREND TOM KEIGHLEY

Reverend Tom Keighley, FRCN, RN, a Hons, DN, RCNT, is an inspirational nurse leader whose main interests are the politics of health care and the challenge of change. In 2001 he established Tom Keighley Associates and began work as an independent health-care consultant. During this time, his skills have been sought by a number of organizations, including the Lincoln Theological Institute and a number of other organizations. He is an international speaker and renowned author.

MAUREEN KELLEY

Maureen Kelley, CNM, PhD, FACNM, is chair of the Family and Community Nursing Department at Emory University's Nell Hodgson Woodruff School of Nursing. She has become increasingly interested in global health and works with the Lillian Carter Center for International Nursing at Emory to develop linkages and partnerships in the Caribbean. She is also a member of the Emory/CDC (Centers for Disease Control) Collaborating Center in Perinatal Health and has worked in perinatal health related to midwifery in Balashikha, Russia.

CAROLE KENNER

Carole Kenner, DNS, RNC, FAAN, is dean and professor of the College of Nursing at the University of Oklahoma. She is past president of the Neonatal Nurses Association and has worked extensively with the World Health Organization on nursing and health-care issues. She received her BSN from the University of Cincinnati, an MSN from Indiana University with a specialty degree in perinatal clinical nurse specialist-CNS/neonatal nurse practitioner, and her doctorate from Indiana University.

SHAKÉ KETEFIAN

Shaké Ketefian, EdD, RN, FAAN, is professor of nursing and director of International Affairs at the University of Michigan School of Nursing. Dr. Ketefian has been a leader in global nursing and established the International Nursing Doctoral Education Network. She is a well-known author and lecturer and is a member of the Expert Panel on Global Nursing and Health.

JO ELLEN KOERNER

Jo Ellen Koerner, PhD, RN, FAAN, is a consultant and founder of the Healing Web, a collaborative education-service model that facilitates service learning in the community. She works in the private sector developing health programs for congregate living communities. She received the Lifetime Achievement Award from American Organization of Nurse Executives in 2005. She is the author of 60 articles and the book *Mother, Heal My Self*, a memoir about her daughter's near-death experience and connecting with a Native American healer.

RUTH ANNE KUIPER

Ruth Anne Kuiper, RN, PhD, CCRN, is associate professor in the School of Nursing at the University of North Carolina at Wilmington. She has been a nurse for 31 years, 17 of which have been in nursing education. Prepared as a clinical specialist in cardiopulmonary nursing with a program of research in self-regulated learning and clinical reasoning, she is an author and speaker at national and international meetings.

RAMÓN LAVANDERO

Ramón Lavandero, RN, MA, MSN, FAAN, is director of development and strategic alliances for the American Association of Critical-Care Nurses (AACN). He is also adjunct associate professor at Indiana University School of Nursing. He was a contributor on the expert panel that developed the AACN Standards for Healthy Work Environments. As former director of the International Leadership Institute at the Honor Society of Nursing, Sigma Theta Tau International, he coordinated planning and the Americas meeting for the honor society's Arista3 conferences. He also served as a faculty member for International Nursing Leadership Institute workshops presented in Russia by the American International Health Alliance.

LINDA LUNA

Linda Luna, RN, PhD, is an international nurse consultant, educator, and executive with 25 years' experience in international settings. She has a diploma, BSN, MSN, and PhD. She also earned a master's of arts in intercultural relations. She has worked internationally in Haiti, Lebanon, Saudi Arabia, and Singapore. She has served on editorial boards of international journals and is a director of the Global Education Development Institute.

SAWSAN ABDUL SALAM MAJALI

Sawsan Abdul Salam Majali, PhD, MSN, BSc, RN, is nursing program director and acting vice dean of student affairs at Dar Al-Hekma College for Girls in Jeddah, Saudi Arabia.

BEVERLY J. MCELMURRY

Beverly J. McElmurry, RN, EdD, FAAN, is assistant dean for global affairs and director and professor of the World Health Organization Collaborating Center for International Development of Primary Health Care at the University of Illinois College of Nursing.

PATRICIA C. MCMULLEN

Patricia C. McMullen, PhD, JD, CNS, CRNP, FNAP, is associate dean for academic affairs at The Catholic University of America School of Nursing. She has combined her interests in nursing and law by conducting research on legal issues in nursing, patient satisfaction with prenatal care, and severe occupational injuries. She has authored a number of research and practice-based articles and texts.

BERNADETTE MAZUREK MELNYK

Bernadette Mazurek Melnyk, PhD, RN, CPNP/NPP, FAAN, FNAP, is dean and Distinguished Foundation Professor of Nursing at Arizona State University College of Nursing, Tempe, Arizona, USA. She is a frequent contributor to the nursing literature and renowned for her work on evidence-based practice.

LYN MIDDLETON

Lyn Middleton, RN, PhD, is coordinator of decentralized mental health nursing programme for the School of Nursing, University of KwaZulu-Natal in Durban, South Africa. She completed her undergraduate and postgraduate work and has been a leader in addressing the issues facing patients with mental health problems.

CHRISTINE O. NEWMAN

Christine O. Newman, MS, RNC, CNNP, is a certified neonatal nurse practitioner and certified regional instructor by the American Academy of Pediatrics and American Heart Association's Neonatal Resuscitation Program. She is a member of the clinical faculty of the neonatal nurse practitioner program at Wayne State University, Detroit, Michigan, USA, and systems administrator for the Henry Ford Hospital neonatal intensive care unit's neonatal database system. She has worked in L'viv, Ukraine, and in Tver, Russia.

ABEL PAIVA

Abel Paiva, MSN, PhD, RN, is medical-surgical specialist at Porto College of Nursing, Porto, Portugal.

MARY PATERSON

Mary Paterson, PhD, RN, is associate professor and assistant dean of undergraduate programs at The Catholic University of America School of Nursing. She has contributed to the design and implementation of primary health-care reform projects in post-conflict, transitional, and developing countries, including Egypt, Jordan, Albania, Iraq, and Russia. Dr. Paterson has a BSN from The Catholic University of America, a master's in nursing administration from Georgetown University, and a PhD in health services and policy analysis with a finance emphasis from the University of California, Berkeley, California, USA.

DANIEL J. PESUT

Daniel J. Pesut, PhD, RN, CS, FAAN, is professor and chair of the Department of Environments for Health at Indiana University. He is past president of Sigma Theta Tau International (2003-05), distinguished lecturer, and recipient of the Edith Moore Copeland Award for Excellence in Creativity in 1993. He is an American Nurses Foundation scholar, a fellow of the American Academy of Nursing, and an honorary fellow of the Amy V. Cockcroft Leadership Development Program.

TIM PORTER-O'GRADY

Tim Porter-O'Grady, DM, EdD, APRN, FAAN, is senior partner, Tim Porter-O'Grady Associates. He has been involved in health care for 37 years and has held roles from staff nurse to senior executive in a variety of health-care settings. He is noted for his work on shared governance models, clinical leadership, conflict, and health futures. He is associate professor and leadership scholar for Arizona State University's Program in Healthcare Innovation. He is also adjunct professor at Lakehead University's School of Public Health in Ontario, Canada.

LARRY PURNELL

Larry Purnell, PhD, RN, FAAN, is a professor in the College of Health Sciences at the University of Delaware. He holds an ADN from Cuyahoga Community College, a BSN from Kent State University, an MSN from Rush University, and a PhD from Columbia Pacific University. His honors include fellowship in the American Academy of Nursing, a Transcultural Scholar, and the Transcultural Nursing Society International Leadership Award. He has more than 100 refereed journal publications, 50 book chapters, and 11 books. His book *Guide to Culturally Competent Health Care* won the AJN Book of the Year Award in 2005. His textbook *Transcultural Healthcare: A Culturally Competent Approach* was awarded the best of the Branden Hill book award in 2003.

DIANNE RICHMOND

Dianne Richmond, RN, MSN, is vice president of clinical excellence for St. Vincent's Health System in Birmingham, Alabama, USA. She completed undergraduate and postgraduate work at the University of Alabama at Birmingham, USA. She has functioned in many clinical roles over the past 30 years.

CYNDA H. RUSHTON

Cynda H. Rushton, PhD, RN, FAAN, is associate professor at Johns Hopkins University School of Nursing in Baltimore, Maryland, USA, and is on the faculty at Johns Hopkins University's Berman Institute of Bioethics. Dr. Rushton is also a clinical nurse specialist in ethics and is program director for the Harriet Lane Compassionate Care Program at Johns Hopkins Children's Center. She is an NIGH international co-director and a 2006 fellow in the Robert Wood Johnson Executive Nurse Fellowship Program. She is a nationally and internationally recognized speaker and consultant.

SHEILA A. RYAN

Sheila A. Ryan, PhD, RN, FAAN, is an endowed professor at the University of Nebraska College of Nursing in Omaha, Nebraska, USA. An internationally recognized leader, consultant, and educator in nursing and health care, she has been a dean for 22 years at two universities and has extensive board service with the Institute of Healthcare Improvement, the American International Health Alliance, the Robert Wood Johnson Foundation, and Institute of Medicine committees. She is a member of the Institute of Medicine. Dr. Ryan earned her BSN from the University of Nebraska, her MSN from the University of California at San Francisco, and her PhD from the University of Arizona.

MARLA E. SALMON

Marla E. Salmon, ScD, RN, FAAN, is dean and professor of the Nell Hodgson Woodruff School of Nursing. She is also the founding director of the Lillian Carter Center for International Nursing and is professor at the Rollins School of Public Health at Emory University, Atlanta, Georgia, USA. She is former director of the Division of Nursing for the U.S. Department of Health and Human Services. She is former chair of the World Health Organization's Global Advisory Group on Nursing and Midwifery and has been a leader in global nursing and health care.

JANE SALVAGE

Jane Salvage, BA, MSc, RGN, HonLLD, is a nurse and independent health consultant with wide experience, particularly in the countries of Central and Eastern Europe and former Soviet Union countries. She is visiting professor of the Florence Nightingale School of Nursing and Midwifery, King's College London, England, and is former director of the European Bureau of the World Health Organization's nursing division.

ELENA STEMPOVSCAIA

Elena Stempovscaia, PhD, RN, is president of the Nursing Association of Moldova. She is a graduate of the International Nursing Leadership Institute and has presented before international nursing audiences. She partners with the Nursing Association of Romania, the Irish Nursing Association, Help Age International, Caritas Moldova, the National Forum of Health Education and Home Care, and the American International Health Alliance.

PAMELA AUSTIN THOMPSON

Pamela Austin Thompson, MS, RN, FAAN, is chief executive officer of the American Organization of Nurse Executives. Prior to that, she was vice president of obstetrics, psychiatric services, and strategic planning at Children's Hospital at Dartmouth, Dartmouth-Hitchcock Medical Center, in Lebanon, New Hampshire, USA. She earned her BSN from the University of Connecticut and her MS from the University of Rochester.

K. JANE YOUNGER

K. Jane Younger, MSN, RN, is president of the Kentucky Nurses Foundation and vice president of the Global Education Development Institute. She served as chief operating officer of Clark Memorial Hospital and chief nursing officer of Jewish Hospital in Louisville, Kentucky, USA. She directed the St. Petersburg-Louisville health-care partnership sponsored by the American International Health Alliance (AIHA), chaired the AIHA International Nursing Task Force, and is a faculty member for the AIHA International Nursing Leadership Institutes.

TABLE OF CONTENTS

FOREWORD

The nursing profession is much like a kaleidoscope—multifaceted, colorful, and constantly taking on different forms and shapes. Like the diversity and creativity seen through a kaleidoscope as one twists and turns it, the nursing career also produces different forms, opportunities, and experiences based on the path that is chosen. The nurse leaders who have contributed to *Nursing Without Borders: Values, Wisdom, Success Markers* have each brought their career kaleidoscope into individual view. Some have chosen to focus their view on administration, education, or research. Others have focused on clinical practice, policy, and system delivery. All, however, have found common ground in their belief in nurses' contributions to global health.

Globalization, international, multinational; collaboration, partnership, alliance—these are all terms that every profession, including nursing, is defining. People in all professions believe these concepts are inherently good and noble, but frequently are unsure about implementation and best practices. *Nursing Without Borders* provides these practices and exemplars.

This masterfully written book allows the reader to look through the kaleidoscopic perspectives of these nurse leaders from diverse cultures around the globe, all working toward diverse outcomes for global health. It is a rare opportunity for readers to learn what each did and share the experience of these leaders in their journey to success. It is an opportunity to see leadership in action. The stories are those of values and wisdom, of trust and community, of methods and practices, and of enrichment and growth. Most of all, the stories are of successes—of impact on institutions, countries, and governments—and of the influence of nurses in making this a healthier world.

There is a remarkable camaraderie in nursing that has no borders. It is formed out of the central desire to make a difference. This book illustrates how nursing leadership has made that difference, has improved the profession, and has impacted the health of people worldwide.

Enjoy these success stories and the glimpses into professional kaleidoscopes. Consider turning and twisting your kaleidoscope to make a similar difference.

—NANCY DICKENSON-HAZARD, RN, MS, FAAN
CHIEF EXECUTIVE OFFICER
HONOR SOCIETY OF NURSING,
SIGMA THETA TAU INTERNATIONAL

INTRODUCTION

Nursing Without Borders: Values, Wisdom, Success Markers reflects the international nursing experiences of a host of nurse leaders representing diverse cultures.

In Part I, several renowned authors address *Values*. They share their experiences and their expertise, setting the tone for learning. The first chapter, written by Sharon M. Weinstein, traces the paths of legendary nursing leaders. We learn that the first nursing license in the world was issued in New Zealand and that leaders from Australia to Ireland and from Jamaica to Italy set the standard by which we now practice, educate, and collaborate. Weinstein effectively transitions us from a proud past to those who are creating nursing's future—the contributors to *Nursing Without Borders*. Barbara M. Dossey, Deva-Marie Beck, and Cynda H. Rushton, leaders of the Nightingale Initiative for Global Health, introduce us to "Nightingale's Vision for Collaboration" in Chapter 2. And, Jane Salvage, visiting professor at the Florence Nightingale School of Nursing and Midwifery, King's College, and former nursing director of the European Bureau for the World Health Organization (WHO), addresses the pleasure and pain of international collaboration. In Chapter 3, she offers sound advice for collaboration and a model for nurses planning to expand their work into the international arena.

In Part II, the authors address *Wisdom*. The wisdom gleaned by nurses from the new independent states of the former Soviet Union (NIS) and Central and Eastern European countries (CEE) is shared through the International Nursing Leadership Institute (INLI) in Chapter 4. Authors Sharon M. Weinstein, Elena Stempovscaia, and K. Jane Younger relate INLI successes and the changes that have been implemented by NIS/CEE nurse leaders. The Honor Society of Nursing, Sigma Theta Tau International played a strong role in inducting INLI graduates into honor society chapters as community leaders. In Chapter 5, Ramón Lavandero, director of development and strategic alliances for the American Association of Critical-Care Nurses (AACN), takes us along the journey to developing standards for establishing and sustaining healthy work environments. And Reverend Tom Keighley, a well-known nurse advocate and lecturer, discusses mutual recognition agreements in Chapter 6.

Part III, focused on *Success Markers*, brings the successes of co-authors Sheila A. Ryan and Majeda Mohammed El-Banna to the forefront in Chapter 7, "Leadership Alliances and Diverse Relationships." The Nebraska-Jordan connection enhances our learning process.

In Chapter 8, Ellen Fineout-Overholt and Bernadette Mazurek Melnyk present "Advancing Evidence-Based Practice in the United States and Across the Globe." They share a 20-year journey that has enabled them to make a difference in outcomes, both at the point of care and in academia. And in Chapter 9, Ann Marie T. Brooks discusses "Creating Communities of International Collaboration," highlighting the work of renowned international nursing leaders and the World Health Organization Collaborating Centers (WHOCC). Brooks skillfully addresses communities of collaboration created through building trust, communicating respect, valuing and celebrating similarities and differences, and sharing knowledge to advance nursing education, practice, and research.

Part IV turns attention to success stories in international nursing. Here we learn about collaborative success from Marjorie Beyers, a nursing consultant who worked with the All-Ukrainian Nursing Association to create a federation model.

Carole Kenner and Anita Finkelman share an effort aimed at "Collaborating for the World's Children: Council of International Neonatal Nurses." Our children are our future, regardless of where we live and work.

Leah Curtin, well-known author and publisher, shares her approach in "War Is Nothing Like You Think. It's Much More!" She relates her experiences in Croatia and shares the creation of the children's book that has garnered international attention.

Pamela Austin Thompson, chief executive officer of the American Organization of Nurse Executives, relates "Process Improvements in Global Health," building on her experience with the American International Health Alliance's partnership program.

Kathleen A. Bower, principal and co-owner of the Center for Case Management, addresses "Nursing as an International Relationship." She highlights her experiences in Barcelona, Spain, and in Singapore. Bower encourages us not to hesitate to accept the opportunity to work with colleagues in other countries, stating that it is an enriching experience that provides many positive memories, even if it is not highly rewarding financially.

"The China Experience" is covered by Beverly J. McElmurry, assistant dean for global affairs and professor and director of the WHO Collaborating Center for International Development of Primary Healthcare at the University of Illinois College of Nursing. Lessons learned through the China Nurses' Leadership Initiative for HIV/AIDS Care and Prevention may be applicable to other international work.

Larry Purnell of the University of Delaware leads us through the Purnell Model for Cultural Competence, and finally, Dianne Richmond, with colleagues Maria Helena Larcher Caliri and Lyn Middleton, share their success with a multinational writing collaborative.

Part V continues our success-story journey with practice experiences. Marianne E. Hess, hospital education coordinator at George Washington University Hospital, shares her experiences in Yerevan, Armenia, following the earthquake and the dissolution of the former Soviet Union. Using adult learning principles, she created an educational model designed to withstand the test of time.

Christine O. Newman, director of neonatal nursing and international partnerships at Henry Ford Health System, writes that "Little Things Really Do Matter." Newman, with colleagues from L'viv, transformed a neonatal unit into a first-class neonatal intensive care unit and offered train-the-trainer programs to support the practice.

Jennifer Andrews and Jeanne M. Floyd, in collaboration with the American Nurses Credentialing Center, share highlights from Princess Alexandra Hospital Health Service District's Magnet journey. Based in Brisbane, Queensland, the hospital achieved Magnet recognition in 2005.

Tim Porter-O'Grady, a renowned consultant and scholar, discusses the transformation of a New Zealand health system and the need to build strong strategic foundations. He shows how strengthening the infrastructure of shared leadership and shared governance helped create a format as well as specific forums for decision-making and accountability.

"A Portuguese Experience With ICNP" is addressed by Abel Paiva of Portugal and co-authors Amy Coenen and Claudia Bartz of the University of Wisconsin, Milwaukee. A standardized model was developed to facilitate pre-coordination of terms, pre-association of nursing diagnoses and nursing interventions, and articulation between the natural language and the standardized language.

Standards determine professional practice, and certification validates expertise in a specific body of knowledge. Mary Alexander, chief executive officer of the Infusion Nurses Society (INS) and the Infusion Nurses Certification Corporation (INCC), is uniquely qualified to address Global Standards and Certification. She discusses her experience at Grupo Angeles' School of Health, supported by the University of Mexico, which is recognized by Mexico's

Ministry of Education. Alexander helped to develop an infusion program for nurses that would provide the knowledge and skills needed to deliver safe, standardized infusion care.

Daniel J. Pesut, with Ruth Anne Kuiper and Carme Espinosa I. Fesnedo, take us along a Network Weaving journey. The authors address the Outcome Present State Test (OPT) Model of reflective clinical reasoning, building on the heritage of the nursing process and the correlation with contemporary needs for outcome specification and attention to clinical judgment.

This part of the book closes with a discussion of migration by Clarita D. Curato and Ma. Katherine O. Jiongco of the Philippines and their U.S. colleague, Jo Ellen Koerner of Adventist Health System. The authors describe a unique model of foreign recruitment and retention that has served both partners well.

We now transition from practice to education and the final series of success stories within Part VI. Rita M. Carty of George Mason University opens this session with "Building a Community of New Scholars." Her story addresses the process and outcomes of 10 years of collaboration, knowledge, and resources incorporated into this international education program in nursing in Saudi Arabia.

Linda Luna and Sawsan Abdul Salam Majali continue the educational partnership series with "A Unique Service-Education Partnership to Advance Nursing in Saudi Arabia." They discuss a collaborative effort between Dar Al-Hekma College and the King Faisal Specialist Hospital and Research Center in Jeddah, Saudi Arabia, aimed at developing and launching a new school of nursing in the western region of the country.

Joyce J. Fitzpatrick of Case Western Reserve University discusses "Success in Preparation of Future Nurse Scientists and Nurse Leaders: A Global Perspective." Through a WHO Collaborating Center, Fitzpatrick impacted thousands of nurses and nursing education in Uganda, Zimbabwe, Ireland, Thailand, and Korea.

Shaké Ketefian of the University of Michigan School of Nursing discusses the International Network for Doctoral Education in Nursing (INDEN) and the creation and subsequent development of the program from its inception to the present.

Global nursing experiences and the opportunity to serve vulnerable communities are the topics of discussion for Maureen Kelley and Marla E. Salmon of Nell Hodgson Woodruff

School of Nursing at Emory University. Theirs is a faith-based initiative, and they worked with the Regional Nursing Body of the Caribbean Community (CARICOM), leading them to the Missionaries of the Poor (MOP) in inner-city Kingston, Jamaica.

Next, Mary Paterson and Patricia C. McMullen of The Catholic University of America share their experiences in Kosovo and Egypt in "International Collaborative Initiatives for Nurses." Through the Hope Fellowship, the authors enhanced educational initiatives and were instrumental in the appointment of the first chief nurse of the Ministry of Health in Kosovo.

The US-Russian Nursing Conference Cruise is an educational model that has received international recognition. Leading this program are authors Marie J. Driever of Portland, Oregon, and Rachel DiFazio of Children's Hospital in Boston. They discuss the US-Russian Nursing Conference Cruise as a catalyst for collaborative professional development.

Finally, we summarize 45-plus years of international nursing leadership in a success story written by Anne J. Davis of the University of California, San Francisco, School of Nursing. Davis takes us through her journey from Ethiopia to India and around the globe, impacting lives along the way. She states that a remarkable camaraderie exists in nursing that is unseen in other professional groups and that there are always those who are willing to help.

And help is precisely what these nurse scholars, educators, researchers, and clinicians have done. As pioneers, they have paved a path of international partnerships and documented their stories for those considering international work.

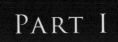

PART I

VALUES

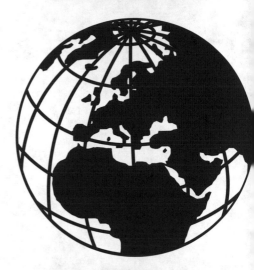

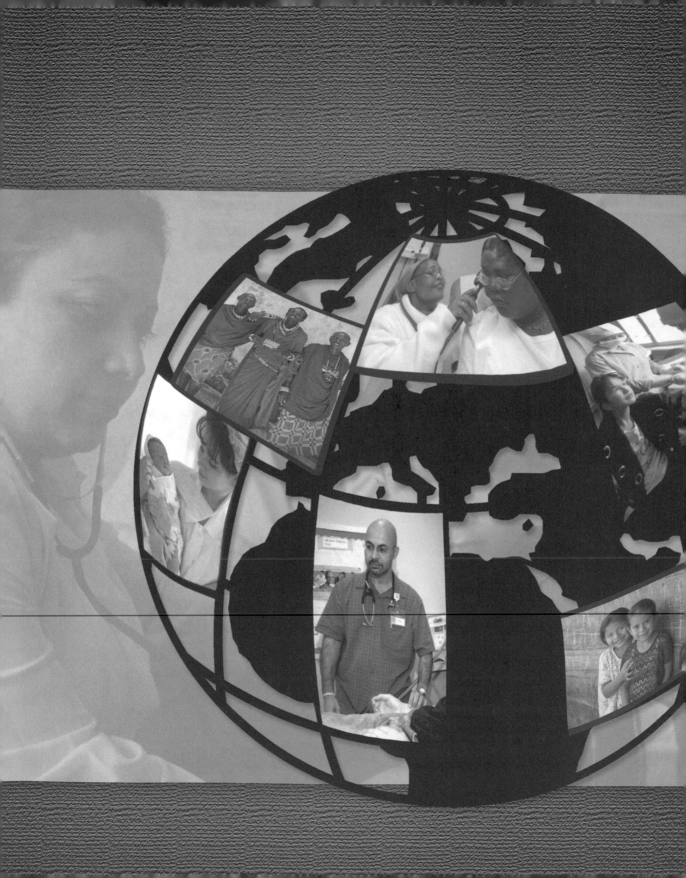

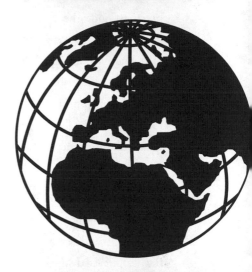

CHAPTER 1

LEGENDARY LEADERS

SHARON M. WEINSTEIN, MS, RN, CRNI, FAAN

The emergence of nursing as a profession occurred in the late 19th century, but the care of children, the sick, the injured, and the wounded has always been instinctive and dates from early history. In 1634 St. Vincent de Paul founded the *Filles de Charite* (Sisters of Charity) to provide training for home visits, hospital experience, and care of the sick. It was not until 1846 that a hospital and school were established in Kaiserwerth, Germany, to provide formal training for nurses. Nursing as a separate profession is not well documented in ancient civilizations. We know that midwives were accepted as specialists in women's health and that priestesses performed functions now recognized as nursing (Donahue, 1996). In 2000 BCE, men, as well as women, functioned as caregivers. Nurses, pharmacists, and physicians were recorded in ancient Greek mythology.

Little mention of hospitals and nursing is made in ancient China, although Halls of Healing are described. One theory about the absence of hospitals in ancient China is that families cared for their own. Within the Christian world, the rise of religious and social movements led to

systematic development of nursing. Care was often provided by deaconesses, widows, Roman matrons, and others. As the 15th century approached its close, we can see the influence of the healing arts. From a world in which military nursing orders carried the chief burden of nursing to the late middle ages, we witness the evolution of nursing. Mid-nineteenth century reforms reshaped the nursing profession, and nursing's early leaders created our present and our future. Let us learn from their lessons; let us share images of legendary leaders from across the globe. These professionals were nursing's pioneers. They set the standard by which we now model ourselves and our practices.

AUSTRALIA
LUCY OSBURN

Lucy Osburn dressed like a nun, wore a cross necklace, and assumed the title Lady Superior; she also aroused suspicion and hostility in a colony already engulfed in religious tensions between Catholics and Protestants. Osburn, the founder of modern nursing in Australia, argued with surgeons, was vilified by the press, became the subject of a Royal Commission, was embroiled in a royal shooting, and ultimately was rejected by her heroine, Florence Nightingale. Osburn's nursing career began at Florence Nightingale's school of nursing in London, and she introduced Nightingale's methods at the Sydney Infirmary (later the Sydney Hospital).

INDIA
BAI KASHIBAI GANPAT

In South India, an edict dated 1097 of Veera Chola Maharaj refers to a 16-bed hospital for students of the district school. Bai Kashibai Ganpat was the first Indian nurse. He was trained in 1891. However, the nursing profession had been brought to India earlier, in 1888, when 10 nursing sisters arrived from England. By 1990, India was home to 23 nursing schools/colleges. The history of India reveals an extensive description of nursing principles and practice; historical documents make reference to nurses, most of whom were men with high standards, skill, and integrity. (Kothare, S.A. & Pai, S.J., n.d.)

IRELAND
CATHERINE MCAULEY

Catherine McAuley's parents died when she was young, and she was adopted as a teenager by a wealthy couple, the Callaghans. At the time of their death, she inherited a substantial property and income that enabled her to build a large residence where she housed orphans and lower income women and cared for them. Her initial goal was to create a group of secular women who would assist with the work. The Catholic Church did not approve, and she was persuaded to form a religious congregation. She entered the Presentation Order with two colleagues and then left to form the Congregation of Mercy in 1831 as a group of *walking sisters* who visited the poor and needy in their places of residence.

With a well-established school, she introduced a modified version of the Lancasterian Monitorial System to her poor schools in Dublin. McAuley's school affiliated with the National Board in 1839. She was a legend in education and health.

MARY AIKENHEAD

Mary Aikenhead was from County Cork. She is most remembered for founding the Congregation of the Irish Sisters of Charity, an order of *walking sisters*, who were free to move outside their convents to serve the poor in hospitals, refuges, and poor schools. St. Vincent's Hospital, Dublin, was founded in 1834, and the congregation made foundations in several places in Ireland and abroad.

ITALY
ST. CAMILLUS DE LELLIS

St. Camillus de Lellis (1550–1614) founded the Nursing Order of Ministers of the sick. Through this order, men cared for the dying, for those stricken with the Black Plague, and alcoholics. St. Camillus de Lellis was born at Bacchianico, Naples, in 1550. He devoted himself to caring for the sick and became director of St. Giacomo Hospital in Rome. As a nurse, he ministered to the sick of Holy Ghost Hospital in Rome, created a larger facility in Naples in 1588, and attended the plague-stricken aboard ships in Rome's harbor and in Rome. In 1591 and 1605, he created the first field medical units when he sent members of his order out to tend wounded troops in Hungary and Croatia. (Catholic Online, n.d.)

JAMAICA
MARY SEACOLE

The pioneering nurse and heroine of the Crimean War, Mary Seacole, was born Mary Jane Grant in 1805 to a Scottish father and a Jamaican mother. Discriminated against because of her color, she learned her nursing skills from her mother who maintained a boarding house for wounded soldiers. Seacole loved to travel, and she visited Haiti, Cuba, and the Bahamas, where she pursued the study of herbal-based medicine to augment European medical ideas. As a result of her service to wounded soldiers, she was awarded the British Crimean medal, the Turkish Medjidie, and the French Legion of Honour.

NATIVE AMERICAN
SUSIE WALKING BEAR YELLOWTAIL

Susie Walking Bear Yellowtail was the first American Indian graduate registered nurse. She completed formal nursing education at the Franklin County Memorial Hospital in Northfield, Massachusetts, and then practiced at Boston City Hospital. In 1978, the American Indian Nurses Association named her *Grandmother of American Indian Nurses*. Born on the Crow Agency reservation in Montana, Susie Walking Bear Yellowtail was not only the first American Indian registered nurse in the United States, but also an activist who fought tirelessly to achieve better health care for Indian people. After graduating from Boston City Hospital School of Nursing in 1923, she returned to Crow Agency to work in the Bureau of Indian Affairs Hospital. The injustices she witnessed there—such as the forced sterilization of Crow women without their consent—galvanized her into a lifelong fight to end abuses in the American Indian health care system.

From 1930 to 1960, the Crow/Sioux nurse traveled to reservations throughout the country to assess the problems American Indians faced. One of Yellowtail's assessments revealed that seriously ill Navajo children were literally dying on the backs of their mothers, who often had to walk 20 miles or more to reach the nearest hospital. To fight these inequities, she joined state health advisory boards and quickly became well known among national healthcare policymakers.

In the 1970s, Yellowtail was appointed to President Nixon's Council on Indian Health, Education, and Welfare and to the federal Indian Health Advisory Committee. These appointments gave her a national platform for advocating for the health needs of her people. She also founded the first professional association for Native American nurses and was instrumental in winning tribal and government funding to help American Indians enter the nursing profession. In 1962, Yellowtail received the President's Award for Outstanding Nursing Health Care.

NEW ZEALAND
ELLEN DOUGHERTY

New Zealand was the first country in the world to regulate nurses nationally, and on January 10, 1902, Ellen Dougherty became the first registered nurse in New Zealand and in the world. The Nurses Registration Act required nurses to train for 3 years and sit for a written examination. During this first year experienced nurses could register without sitting for an examination.

Dougherty was employed by the Wellington District Hospital, completed a certificate in nursing in 1887, and studied elementary anatomy and physiology. She became head of the hospital's accident ward and also ran the surgery ward. (Openshaw, 2006)

A nursing museum located in the Auckland War Memorial Museum in Auckland, New Zealand, is home to *100 Years of Nursing* and focuses on the people behind the uniform and their roles as pioneers in nursing. The collection includes photos of nurses in Russia and from the "First Fifty" nurses to leave New Zealand for World War I in 1915.

PHILIPPINES
ANASTACIA GIRON TUPAS

Filipinos are a diverse group both racially and culturally, including the descendants of aborigines as well as of Indonesians, Malays, Chinese, Japanese, and Spanish who intermarried; they speak a total of 87 languages. Spanish and American colonization of the Philippines significantly affected healthcare delivery. Hospitals were established by Spanish colonial administrators. Missionaries and religious men known as *hospitallers* provided nursing care. Philippine male attendants were trained by the missionaries to help with nursing care. Anastacia Giron Tupas was founder of the Philippine Nurses Association (PNA). PNA now has 92 local chapters; 9 international chapters (America, Austria, Australia, Norway, Switzerland, United Kingdom, Malaysia, Saudi Arabia, and Singapore); and is a member of the International Council of Nurses.

During the Philippine-American War from 1899 to 1902, women with no formal nursing training volunteered to take care of wounded Philippine soldiers. They dressed wounds and provided physical and psychological aid to the sick. The earliest nursing schools were found in Visaya and Luzon. The first college of nursing or nursing program was the University of Santo Tomas in 1944; the college itself was founded in 1611.

RUSSIA

VALENTINA IVANOVNA CHEBOTAREVA

Valentina Ivanovana Chebotareva served in the military hospital in Tsarskoye Selo, Russia, during World War I. Tschebotarioff (1964), writes that Chebotareva had volunteered as a nurse earlier during the Russo-Japanese War of 1904–1905 and had formal nursing training at the time. Even though she was not in the highest of social circles, she did work with the Tsarina and her daughters. Chebotareva continued her volunteer hospital work until 1919, when she died of typhus. She was honored posthumously when her son, Gregory, was given a ribbon by her fellow nurses that read, "From the Trustees and the Army Hospitals to the unforgettable V. I. Chebotareva who gave her life 'for her friends.'"

TATIANA NIKOLAIEVNA ROMANOVA

Tatiana Nikolaievna Romanova headed Red Cross committees during World War I. With her mother and sister, she cared for wounded soldiers in a private hospital on the grounds of Tsarskoye Selo. She was considered a skilled caregiver; although because of her youth, she was spared many of the more trying cases.

GRAND DUCHESS HELENA PAVLOVNA

During the Crimean War, the Grand Duchess Helena Pavlovna and her Sisters of Mercy of the Community of the Cross were nursing Russian soldiers (Sorokina, 1995). Nursing in Russia during the Tsarist era had no infrastructure. Typical nurses of the 19th century were "Sisters of Mercy," working within the communities of the Orthodox Church and religious societies to provide a military nursing service. Following the war, the body of knowledge and experience did not transfer throughout the regions, and many of Russian's citizens received inadequate medical and little nursing care.

SOUTH KOREA
PROFESSOR MO-IM KIM

Perhaps one of Korea's most distinguished nursing leaders, Professor Mo-Im Kim was the first woman in the Republic of South Korea to lead a government ministry and the first non-physician to be appointed Minister of Health (MOH). Active in the International Council of Nurses (ICN) and the World Health Organization (WHO), she received many honors and awards. In 1994, she was awarded the Sasakawa Prize in Health by the WHO along with a substantial cash prize. This award facilitated the creation of the Kim-Sasakawa Fund to support reunification of nursing in Korea. Yonsei University has played a significant role in history since its inception in the early 1900s and has been the site of many professional exchanges on a global scale.

TURKEY
MADAME ANTONIETTE

Modern nursing is said to have had its birth in the country that is today known as Turkey. In 1854, Britain and France, responding to invasion of the Ottoman Empire by Russia, came to the empire's aid in the Crimean War. Students of nursing are well aware of Florence Nightingale's important role in caring for British soldiers involved in that war, but she was not the first to introduce modern nursing practices to this area. In 1820—more than 30 years before Nightingale's arrival in Anatolia, also known as Asia Minor—American missionaries brought improvements in nursing practice to this region. In 1842, female students were able to enroll in medical school courses for training in midwifery. Ten female nurses received graduate certificates in 1845, nearly a decade before the Crimean War.

Following the Crimean War, national and international foundations evolved in support of adequate healthcare for all. 1868, the Ottoman Empire established a foundation in Istanbul called *Hilal-i Ahmer*. Founded by 50 members, 10 of whom were women, the organization provided care and education to the injured, operating on the principle that "we are all siblings." Women played important roles in providing care to the poor (Behmoaras, 2001).

Beginning with the First and Second Balkan Wars (1912–13), continuing through the First World War (1913–18) and the Turkish War of Independence (1919–22), and culminating with the Treaty of Lausanne in 1923, women offered help to the sick and wounded. Effective training was a primary concern; one of the caregivers was Madame Antoniette, the wife of a chief physician. She volunteered as a nurse's aide during the Balkan Wars (Akgün and Ulugtekin, 2000).

UNITED STATES
FRAY (FRIAR) JUAN DE MENA

Juan de Mena was shipwrecked off of the south Texas Coast nearly 70 years prior to the landing of the Pilgrims. He is the first identified nurse in what became the United States. He created a charity to tend the sick. He was Mexico's nurse, esteemed and praised for his diligence until the time he was deceived, along with others, into leaving his province for Spain and was led to his death (Skally, 2002).

VIRGINIA HENDERSON

Virginia Henderson has been described as the *first lady of nursing*. An accomplished author, an avid researcher, and a visionary, she is considered by many to be the most important nursing figure in the 20th century. A respected leader, she made significant and lasting contributions to the nursing profession, including a definition of nursing with sufficient precision and poetry to become the internationally adopted statement of who we are; three of the *Principles and Practice of Nursing* that elaborated on the knowledge base necessary to act in terms of the definition; a survey and an assessment of nursing research that shifted nursing research away from studying nurses to studying the differences that nurses can make in people's lives; and the *Nursing Studies Index* that captured the intellectual history of the first 6 decades of the 20th century. An internationally recognized leader, she was the recipient of numerous awards including the prestigious first Christiane Reimann Prize, recognizing that her span of influence knew no national boundaries. Sigma Theta Tau International's nursing library bears her name (Abrams, 2007).

HILDEGARD PEPLAU

A leading nurse, theorist, and the mother of psychiatric nursing, Dr. Hildegard Peplau led the field. The only nurse to serve the America Nurses Association as executive director and later as President, she was also elected to serve two terms on the Board of the International Council of Nurses (ICN). In 1997 she received the world of nursing's highest honour, the Christiane Reimann Prize, at the ICN Quadrennial Congress. This award is given once every 4 years for outstanding national and international contributions to nursing and healthcare. In 1996, the American Academy of Nursing named her a "Living Legend," and in 1998 the American Nurses Association (ANA) inducted her into the ANA Hall of Fame.

Dr. Peplau's book, *Interpersonal Relations in Nursing* (1952), was completed in 1948. At that time, it was unusual for a nurse to publish a book without a physician co-author; thus, publication was delayed for 4 years. Internationally recognized for her contributions to the profession, she has revolutionized nursing practice and education.

MARGRETTA MADDEN STYLES

Margretta Madden Styles served global nursing as president of the American Nurses Association, the International Council of Nurses, and the American Nurses Credentialing Center; she was perhaps one of nursing's most influential and respected leaders.

Styles was responsible for the development of several schools of nursing from inception, including the University of Texas, San Antonio. She served as dean at Wayne State and the University of California, San Francisco. Her career and her commitment took her across the country and around the globe. A leader of Credentialing International and efforts to engage foreign nursing programs within the Magnet initiative, Styles will long be remembered as the ultimate professional, a visionary leader with a passion for educational administration, professional organization development, and credentialing. She has left an amazing mark on the profession and on those whose lives she touched.

PAST, PRESENT, AND FUTURE

In the beginning, there was a vision, one that became a reality. First, we had nursing's legendary leaders stemming from all corners of the globe. These leaders set the stage for the growth of the profession and the professionals. We have shared some of nursing's global pioneers and their stories with you. *Nursing Without Borders* is a format for introducing leaders of this generation to the next generation of leaders. These professionals represent the present and the future—a future of which each nurse is a significant part (Jennings, 2002). Peter Drucker once said, "The best way to predict the future is to create it." These stories demonstrate that the contributors look *beyond borders* with a vision like that of the legendary leaders whose paths they follow. They are creating nursing's future through global partnerships that will continue to flourish and impact future generations of nurses. The impact of this work will reach far into the next century and will serve as a foundation upon which even greater advancements may develop. Nurses, nursing, and society at large will benefit.

REFERENCES

Akgün, S.K. & Ulugtekin, M. (2000). *Hilal-i* Ahmer'den Kizilay'a. Ankara: Beyda Basimevi.

Abrams, S. (2007). Nursing the community, a look back at the 1984 dialogue between Virginia A. Henderson and Sherry L. Shamansky. *Public Health Nursing*, Volume 24, Number 4, July/August 2007, pp. 382-386(5).

Behmoaras, L. (2001). *Mazhar Osman, Kapali kutudaki firtina* 3. Baski Istanbul, Remzi Kitabevi s. 232.

Catholic Online. (n.d.). St. Camillus de Lellis. Retrieved 2 October 2007 from http://www.catholic.org/saints/saint.php?saint_id=265.

Donahue, M. (1996). *Nursing: The finest art* (2nd ed.) St. Louis, MO. Mosby.

Jennings, C. (2002). Nurses must create the future they want. *Policy, Politics, & Nursing Practice*, Vol. 3, No. 4, 287-288 (2002). DOI: 10.1177/152715402237439.

Kothare, S.N. & Pai, S.A. (n.d.). *An introduction to the history of medicine.* Retrieved 2 October 2007 from http://www.histmedindia.org/.

Openshaw, M., (2007). Dougherty, Ellen 1844–1919. *Dictionary of New Zealand Biography*. Updated 22 June 2007. Retrieved 2 October 2007 from http://www.dnzb.govt.nz/.

Skally, R. (2002). *Career series: Men in nursing gain respect as attitudes change*

Sorokina, T. (1995). Russian nursing in the Crimean War. *Journal of the Royal College of Physicians of London, 29* (1), 57–61.

Tschebotarioff, G. P. (1964). *Russia: My native land: A U.S. engineer reminisces and looks at the present.* McGraw-Hill Book Company, ASIN B00005XTZJ, 244. Retrieved from http://en.wikipedia.org/wiki/Valentina_Ivanovna_Chebotareva.

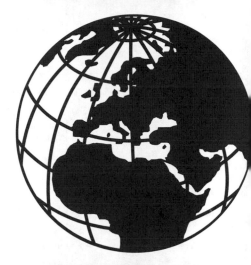

CHAPTER 2

NIGHTINGALE'S VISION FOR COLLABORATION

BARBARA M. DOSSEY, PhD, RN, AHN-BC, FAAN,
DEVA-MARIE BECK, PhD, RN,
CYNDA H. RUSHTON, PhD, RN, FAAN

The Nightingale Initiative for Global Health (NIGH) is a nurse-driven initiative aimed at replicating Florence Nightingale's vision among nurses of the world, as well as today's plethora of midwives, professional and allied healthcare team members, other health workers, and concerned citizens. Why Nightingale? Why Now? Why NIGH?

The critical reason is that your family's health, your health, everyone's health is at risk. On Nightingale's birthday on May 12, 2007, the first global nursing Internet signature project, the Nightingale Declaration Campaign (NDC) was launched. We acknowledge that nurses are essential to the creation of a healthy world and that, unless the nursing community is sustained in innovative ways, worldwide, the health of everyone on the planet will be in serious jeopardy. See Figure 2.1, Nightingale Declaration of Commitment for Healthy World by 2020.

"We, the nurses and concerned citizens of the global community, hereby dedicate ourselves to achieve a healthy world by 2020. We declare our willingness to unite in a program of action, to share information and solutions and to improve health conditions for all humanity—locally, nationally, and globally. We further resolve to adopt personal practices and to implement public policies in our communities and nations—making this goal achievable and inevitable by the year 2020, beginning today in our own lives, in the life of our nations and in the world at large."

Signature_____

Figure 2.1. *Nightingale Declaration of Commitment for a Healthy World by 2020.*

(http://www.nightingaledeclaration.net)

Source: © Nightingale Declaration of Commitment for a Healthy World by 2020. (2007) Used with permission of the Nightingale Initiative for Global Health. Available at http://www.nightingaledeclaration.net

Florence Nightingale (1820–1910), the founder of modern nursing, had a clear vision of nurses' key role in promoting health and well-being for all humanity and for future generations: "In the future which I shall not see, for I am old, may a better way be opened! May the methods by which every infant, every human being will have the best chance at health—the methods by which every sick person will have the best chance at recovery be learned and practiced" (Nightingale, 1893).

Unfortunately, Nightingale's dreams are at risk. Today, 80% of the world's healthcare is delivered by nurses and midwives (WHO, 2006). A severe nursing shortage—throughout the

United States (US), Canada, Europe, the rest of the developed world as well as in all developing countries—is creating serious and increasingly-adverse impacts on human health and well-being everywhere (ICN, 2004).

NIGH's collective goal of two million signatures cannot be accomplished without collaboration among nurses. Together, we can realize Nightingale's dreams, making sustainable, compassionate care and healthy lives a birthright—from local to global, around the world. This chapter shares the evolving NIGH story and the development of the NDC.

THE NIGH STORY

Nightingale left a lasting legacy—raising standards for millions of dedicated health professionals who have followed her example through education and training and with multi-skilled devotion to caring for others. Yet, in our demanding preparation for a professional lifetime of caring, few have realized our contemporary need for the additional skills and commitment Nightingale also possessed: the ability to communicate so effectively with others—nurses, colleagues, and the general public—around the globe. Nightingale, the tireless networker, raised awareness of how human health needs anywhere ultimately affect the health of all; she referred to this as "nursing."

The NIGH quest is to fulfill Nightingale's definition that "[h]ealth is not only to be well, but to use well, every power we have"(Nightingale, 1893). It is also to address the following local-to-global questions: How do we make the global community a beautiful and happy place of healthy people? How can the differences and divisions among us become less and the cooperation and collaboration become more, the global conflict diminished and worldwide consensus built towards a common future of health and prosperity for all? How can we work together for a healthy world? And, the key question for everyone to ask themselves personally, what is your calling? We asked ourselves the same questions, and our foundational principles evolved. As we asked ourselves this series of questions, we birthed and nurtured the NIGH and the foundational principles found in Table 2.1.

TABLE 2.1.   FOUR GUIDING PRINCIPLES.

	Focus	Recognition	Impact	Outcome
1	Nursing starts With "I"	Interior "I" space. Experiences, personal meaning, fears, emotions, memories, and esteem.	Brought NIGH team together. Nursing is quiet, individual work. Awareness of "I." Nursing is art.	Cognizant of role in building a healthy world.
2	Nursing is built on "We"	"We" space. Share collective stories, values, meanings, vision, language, and cultural background to create a healthy world.	Called upon to "be with" difficult human experiences. Sense of "We" supports us to recognize suffering.	Increased awareness of relational aspects. New identity in suffering through new meaning. New sense of past. Shift in one's consciousness.
3	"It" is about behavior and skill development.	Importance of individual exterior "It" space.	Cross-cultural understanding, advocacy, and communications embedded in nursing practice worldwide. Train the trainers. Sustaining renewal, resilience, and retention.	Decent care for all.
4	"Its" systems and structures.	Exterior Collective "Its" space with team members and others. Social systems, networks, information technology, and environment.	Further capacity building for national and global arenas.	

PRINCIPLES

NIGH's four foundational principles are based upon Nightingale's vision and her own work that she referred to as "her must." Her legacy, work, and the scope of her lifetime achievements offered a road map. However, we are also charting our contemporary road map; we are striving to be integrally informed in our efforts, partnerships, and collaborations to address healing, leadership, and global action. We believe that nursing can be empowered in innovative ways if nurses around the world feel connected to each other and realize that sincere efforts are being made to increase all aspects of a healthy nursing community and workforce.

BOX 2.1. INTEGRAL MODEL AND FOUR QUADRANTS.

UPPER-LEFT (UL) SUBJECTIVE

The upper-left quadrant highlights the world of the individual interior experiences: thoughts, emotions, memories, perceptions, immediate sensations, and states of mind — imagination, fears, feelings, beliefs, values, esteem, cognitive capacity, emotional maturity, moral development, and spiritual maturity. This is referred to as our "I" space.

UPPER-RIGHT (UR) OBJECTIVE

The upper-right quadrant highlights the world of one individual, exterior things: our material body (physiology [cells, molecules, neurotransmitters, limbic system], biochemistry, chemistry, physics), skill development (health, fitness, exercise, nutrition, etc.), behaviors, practices, patient-care plans, and anything that we can touch or observe scientifically in time and space. This is referred to as the "It" space.

LOWER-LEFT (LL) INTERSUBJECTIVE

The lower-left quadrant highlights the world of our collective, interior experiences: shared values, meanings, vision, language, relationships, and cultural background. This is referred to as the "We" space.

LOWER-RIGHT (LR) INTEROBJECTIVE

The lower-right quadrant highlights the world of the collective, exterior things: social systems/structures; networks; organizational structures and systems (in healthcare, this includes financial and billing systems); information technology; regulatory structures (environmental and governmental policies, etc.); and the natural environment. This is referred to as the "Its" space.

Source: Wilber, K. (2000b). *Integral Psychology: Consciousness, Spirit, Psychology, Therapy*. Boston: Shambhala. Figure adapted with permission from Ken Wilber.

BOX 2.2.   SUFFERING, MORAL SUFFERING, MORAL DISTRESS, AND SOUL PAIN.

Suffering: An individual's story around pain where the signs of suffering may be physical, mental, emotional, social, behavioral, and/or spiritual; it is anguish experienced—internal and external—as a threat to one's composure, integrity, and the fulfillment of intentions.

Moral suffering: Occurs when an individual experiences tensions or conflicts about what is the right thing to do in a particular situation; it often involves the struggle of finding a balance between competing interest or values.

Moral distress: Occurs when an individual is unable to translate moral choices into moral actions and when prevented by obstacles, either internal or external, from acting upon it.

Soul pain: The experience of an individual who has become disconnected and alienated from the deepest and most fundamental aspects of one's self.

Source: Halifax. J., Dossey. B. M., & Rushton, C. H. (2007). *Compassionate Care of the Dying*. Santa Fe, NM: Prajna Mountain Press. Adapted from Jameston, A. (1984). *Nursing practice, the ethical issues*. Englewood Cliffs, NJ: Prentice Hall, and Kearney, M. (1996). *Mortally wounded*. New York: Scribner.

Nightingale was an integralist; her worldview focused on the individual and the collective, the inner and the outer, the human and the nonhuman, as illustrated in Boxes 2.1 (Wilber, 2000, Dossey, 2007 and 2008) and 2.2 (Halifax, Dossey, and Rushton, 2007). Throughout her career, she contributed her unique nursing worldview to care for the individual nurse as well as for the collective endeavors of all healthcare team members and concerned citizens of her time. She frequently demonstrated skills and behaviors that would impact healthcare delivery. She introduced healthcare systems/structures that would transform the health of the world.

The NDC reflects our vision of her dream. These visions call for new interdisciplinary dialogues and a new spirit of creativity and inspiration, commitment and courage, exploration and understanding. NIGH principles reflect how nursing can become more integrally informed to keep nursing sustainable. We continue to "connect the dots" of our diverse experiences—to more deeply understand who we are and how we are related to all of life—local to global—in our partnerships and collaborations.

Ken Wilber offered inspiration through the Integral Model developed more than 30 years ago (Wilber, 1999, 2000a, 2000b). See Figure 2.2. A circle of healing healing has been added at the center, representing an integral and a holistic perspective of nursing (Dossey, Selanders, Beck & Attewell, 2005, Dossey, 2008a and 2008b). Deep inside the circle, these four key words have been placed: "I" (the inside of the individual), "We" (the inside of the collective), "It" (the outside of the individual), and "Its" (the outside of the collective). These represent realities that are already part of our everyday language and awareness. The dotted horizontal and vertical lines illustrate that each quadrant can be understood as permeable and porous, with each quadrant's experiences integrally informing and empowering all other quadrant experiences. Building upon Wilber's Integral Model, we created four principles that encompass the collaborators—all interdisciplinary team members and concerned citizens who joined the NDC. Our NIGH and NDC endeavors address the importance of a local-to-global advocacy strategy for peer support; it also includes media and communications capacity building for the nursing community to raise their voices about how systems and structures can focus on decent care. Figure 2.3 shows a Nightingale quote in each quadrant.

The World Health Organization (WHO, 2008) calls for "decent care" for HIV/AIDS patients and their families throughout the world. The primary objective is to delineate a new term within the taxonomy and politics of HIV/AIDS care—decent care—that repositions the individual as the focal point of the care cycle that emphasizes what type or kind of care individuals receive, but also how that care is received. Decent care implies the comprehensive ideal that the medical, physiological, psychological, and spiritual needs of others are addressed. This includes universal access to treatment with utilization and enforcement of universally accepted precautionary measures for healthcare practitioners, along with adequate supplies and equipment, safe food, free access to clean water, autoclaves, laundries, and safe methods for sterilizing and disposing of infected materials in incinerators.

Nightingale carried more than a literal candlelight to her nightshift rounds in the cavernous halls of a wartime hospital. She also focused on the external structure and systems of all hospital barracks and hospitals where the needs of wounded soldiers were addressed—needs beyond clean dressings and linens and nourishing food. We are all familiar with her work and her unique communication skills. In her time, she was a best-selling author of *Notes on Nursing*, initially written first for a general audience (Nightingale, 1860).

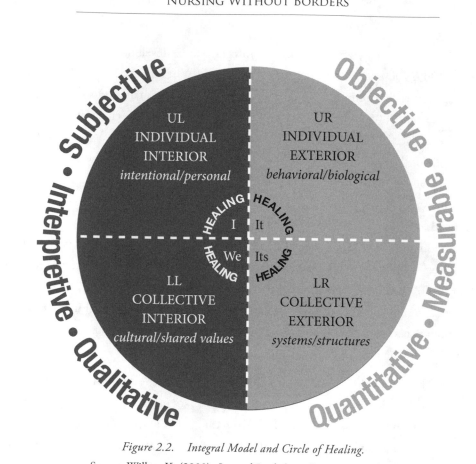

Figure 2.2. Integral Model and Circle of Healing.

Source: Wilber, K. (2000). *Integral Psychology: Consciousness, Spirit,
Psychology, Therapy.* Boston: Shambhala. Figure adapted with
permission from Ken Wilber. (http://www.kenwilber.com) by
Barbara M. Dossey © 2007.

We know that nurses are acclaimed the most trusted professional group in the world. We understand that nurses, midwives, and professional and allied healthcare team members are educated and prepared—physically, emotionally, mentally, and spiritually—to effectively address the activities required on the ground for the health of people. We see the NIGH four principles as a valuable support system, strengthening our endeavors to keep this nursing community sustainable. We consciously use the integral process as a framework to reflect and act upon Nightingale's mandate—a commitment to human health of individuals, of communities, and the world—as a first priority. As we do this, we see that nursing's commitment to human health is more highly respected, appreciated, and valued worldwide.

Nightingale's "Integral" Ideas

Subjective "I"

"Nursing work must be quiet work—An individual work—Anything else is contrary to the whole realness of the work. Where am I, the individual, in my utmost soul? What am I, the inner woman, called "I"?—That is the question." (1888)

Objective "It"

"When we obey all God's laws as to cleanliness, fresh air, pure water, good habits, good dwellings, good drains, food and drink, work and exercise, health is the result: when we disobey, sickness… No epidemic can resist thorough cleanliness and fresh air." (1876)

"Let us run the race where all may win: rejoicing in their successes, as our own and mourning their failures, wherever they are, as our own. We are all one Nurse… The very essence of all good organizations is, that everybody should do her [and his] own work in such a way as to help & not hinder every one else's work." (1873)

"Nursing takes a whole life to learn. We must make progress in it every year…. Nursing is not an adventure, as some have now supposed…. It is a very serious, delightful thing, like life, requiring training, experience, devotion not by fits and starts, patience, a power of accumulating, instead of losing all these things. We are only on the threshold of training." (1897)

Intersubjective "We"

Interobjective "Its"

Figure 2.3. Nightingale Integral. © 2007 NIGH.

RELATIONSHIP BUILDING: CREATING A CONTEMPORARY NIGHTINGALE TEAM

In the 1990s, holistic nursing pioneer Dr. Barbara Dossey joined with Dr. Deva-Marie Beck to craft an integral perspective to focus on sharing Nightingale's phenomenal work with a contemporary global audience. Dossey and Beck recognized a need to move beyond simply describing Nightingale's panoramic life in books and articles. They led a grassroots-to-global initiative to strategically address the health needs of our time, both at home and abroad. They knew that to fully understand how and what Nightingale accomplished in her time contemporary people would need an experience that reached far beyond reading her personal history.

They envisioned an innovative action project that would fully follow in Nightingale's footsteps to seek to improve the health of humanity—not just at local levels, but at regional, national, and global levels as well. The project could demonstrate how nurses can unite in addressing critical global challenges with their coordinated local actions. It could also bring attention to nurses' knowledge, skills, and caring and unite them as "21st-century Nightingales" with each other and for the world. With a focus on the unprecedented global nursing shortage, Dossey, Beck, and Rushton in collaboration with the NIGH team, envisioned featuring nursing's profound value to the health of humanity. Table 2.2 details the timeline of their efforts.

TABLE 2.2.   TIMELINE OF NIGH EVENTS.

Year	Achievement
2002	Initial discussions and founding of the NIGH.
2003	Multidisciplinary collaboration and signature campaign and resolutions.
	Legal counsel appointed.
	Identified international advisory council members.
2004	Identification of initial co-collaborators.
	A service commemorating Florence Nightingale, nurses, and nursing, May 9th, Washington National Cathedral, Washington, D.C., by NIGH team with representatives from the American Association of Nurse Executives, Sigma Theta Tau International, and the National Student Nurses Association.
2005	International plan launched.
	Publication of *Florence Nightingale Today: Healing, Leadership, Global Action*, an *American Journal of Nursing* Book of the Year.
	Active discussions with other global partners.
	Appointment of Cynda H. Rushton as co-director.
	Integral Model, process, and plans for the United Nation's Decade for a Healthy World
	Creation of web site: http://www.nighcommunities.org.
2006	Participated in WHO Global Forum for Chief Nursing and Midwifery Officers.
2006	Don deSilva joins team as information technology strategist.
	Additional list of international advisory council members announced.
2007	UN General Assembly Resolutions slated for November 2008.
	May 12th launch of NDC, and sponsorship program. (www.nightingaledeclaration.net)
	Panel presentation made to Turkish National Student Nurses Congress.
	NDC meeting with Turkish support.
	Presentations to nursing leaders in South America and Asia.

Year	Future Plans
2008–2010	Action plans will be implemented.
	Preparation for 2010 International Year of the Nurse.
2010	International Year of the Nurse and global celebration.
2011–2020	NDC coaching for integral change with local to global workshops.
	Development of related communities of practice.
	Coaching for integral change companion guides will be released in print, CD-ROM, and for iPod format with electronic media tools available.

During this entire period, to further the NIGH vision, mission, mandate, and goals, an evolving strategic 15-year plan has also been articulated. Hence, a non-profit organization based in Washington, D.C. was established as the first of many related NIGH networks envisioned to eventually circle the globe.

The NIGH has received initial funding—all from private donors—totaling in excess of $50,000 and more than 5,000 in-kind hours of professional skills amounting to more than $100,000 in donated services. NIGH has also received generous in-kind support from countless volunteer hours to coordinate logistics at the many meetings noted earlier in this chapter. Extensive contributions of supplies and human capital have led to the success thus far.

COLLABORATING WITH INITIAL SPONSORS AND FUTURE SPONSORS

Building upon all of these efforts and achievements, NIGH circulated the *NDC Concept Paper* to describe the scope and plans and to establish the following sponsorships levels: Platinum Sponsorship at $10,000 and up; Gold Sponsorship from $5,000–$9,999; and Silver Sponsorship from $1,000–$4,999. Corporate benefactors were also added.

As of October, 2008, the NIGH has received platinum sponsorship from the American Nurses Association, Sigma Theta Tau International, and American Association of Critical-Care Nurses. Gold sponsorship has been received from The Johns Hopkins University School of Nursing, the University of Maryland School of Nursing, Indiana University School of Nursing, and the Registered Nurses Association of Ontario. Silver sponsorship has been received from the University of Minnesota School of Nursing, Baylor University Louise Herrington School of Nursing, York University School of Nursing in Toronto, and Dr. Jean Watson. The first corporate silver sponsor is Johnson & Johnson's Campaign for Nursing's Future.

ONGOING ACTIVITIES

As stated by WHO Chief Nursing Scientist, Jean Yan, "nurses add essential value to health care throughout the world. They are catalysts for health development; conveners of nursing leadership groups; collectors of relevant evidence; planners; [and] implementers. While [they have been] often assumed to merely be the 'arms and legs' of health care—nurses are indeed the 'brains and heart' of health care implementation and central to advancing the health of humanity" (WHO, 2006).

However, since Nightingale's time, nursing has most often focused at the "micro" implementation of their core values. This focus has been on external factors, such as delivering healthcare technology, implementing patient/client care plans, and evaluating hospital and healthcare systems and structures. Much less emphasis has been placed on supportive care of the individual nurse and on the value of dialogue to foster understanding between nurses themselves and with other disciplines. A gap between what nurses contribute and what nurses need for this contribution to remain sustainable has continued to widen throughout recent decades. Paying particular attention to the increasingly severe global nursing shortage, the NIGH team has noted that current approaches have been insufficient to create the change necessary to provide optimal patient care, create a healthy work environment, and sustain caregivers in their caregiving roles.

The NIGH process has included a growing awareness that people long for opportunities to be understood, to tell their stories to others who can deeply listen with appreciation and compassion. We recognize that wherever we live and work, we will find others who are quite different from ourselves in culture, creed, and race. Nursing practice traditionally addresses these issues for patients and families. However, nurses are less likely to consider the need to turn appreciatively to each other with the same mind and heart. Thus, NIGH has clarified the need to foster cross-cultural understanding and even nurse-to-nurse diplomacy, particularly as we seek to build a global network of nurses who can support and empower each other on a worldwide scale. This represents the "We" component of the Integral Model.

Lastly, the NIGH team has noted that while nurses are very good at informing each other about maintaining quality nursing practice, nurses have not yet mastered the art of advocating for ourselves and sharing the innate value of nursing's contribution to the world (Buresh and Gordon, 2000). NIGH's own process has included developing dialogue with multimedia and communications professionals to discover how multimedia-capacities can also become imbedded in 21st-century nursing practice. This is particularly needed given the worldwide trend for everyone to achieve new levels of media literacy. The "It" component of the Integral Model calls for developing new media advocacy skills, and the "Its" component of the Integral Model calls for the need to explore beyond nursing's current disciplinary boundaries, especially when an increasingly globalized world sets the pace for what nurses need to contribute with our articulate voices.

THE LAUNCH

An initial key result of the NIGH initiative has been the creation of a global signature campaign for everyone—nurses, midwives, all health professionals and allied healthcare team members, and concerned citizens throughout the world. Based on this grassroots-to-global commitment, NIGH's further goal is to achieve the passage of two United Nations Resolutions (UNRs) for adoption by the UN General Assembly of 2008 to launch (a) 2010: International Year of the Nurse [Centennial of Nightingale's death]; (b) 2011–2020: UN Decade for a Healthy World [Bicentennial of Nightingale's birth, 2020]; and (c) the design and development of Train-the-Trainer Workshops to coincide with the UNRs proposed for passage in 2008.

CHALLENGES

NIGH's challenges continue to be in creating strong partnerships based upon processes and innovations. While we have occasional onsite meetings, most of NIGH's team members and collaborators participate together via telephone and e-mail. This has required significant attention to understanding each other and each other's diverse perspectives across the miles, continents and oceans as though we were actually together face-to-face.

BOX 2.3.   UN MILLENNIUM DEVELOPMENT GOALS AND TARGETS.

1. Eradicate extreme poverty and hunger
2. Achieve universal primary education
3. Promote gender equality and empower women
4. Reduce child mortality
5. Improve maternal health
6. Combat HIV/AIDS, malaria, and other diseases
7. Ensure environmental sustainability
8. Develop global partnerships for development

Source: World Health Organization (2002). WHO Assembly Report: Millennium Development Goals and Targets. Retrieved April 1, 2007, at http://www.who.int/mdg/en and http://www.un.org/millenniumgoals/

NIGH's work to create the NDC and the two UNR proposals also engages us in the global commitment to achieve the eight 2000 UN Millennium Development Goals (MDGs) as seen in Box 2.3 (United Nations, 2000). Three of these issues, Number 4 (child mortality), Number 5 (maternal health), and Number 6 (HIV/AIDS and other diseases), are specifically related to health. Four others, Number 1 (poverty and hunger), Number 2 (primary education), Number 3 (gender equality and empowerment of women), and Number 7 (environmental sustainability), also impact upon human health.

NIGH has also been challenged to discover how best to bring our own integral processes to a wider group of colleagues interested in further collaboration. Despite the magnitude of this challenge, we believe that these learning opportunities can support the more than 80% of the worldwide healthcare workforce that are nurses and midwives and who currently are so significantly at risk across the globe.

Fundraising is likewise a challenge. We are confident that we will attract the funds needed to succeed as we continue to strengthen our stand for the mission and the vision that will draw the necessary resources. Our work and mission have increased our clarity of purpose, authenticity, and boldness as we seek new partnerships. We are also challenged to stay steady and to take good care of ourselves and each other along the way, as this work is very demanding and rewarding.

OUTCOMES AND SUSTAINABILITY

The NIGH and NDC endeavors have already begun to demonstrate that consensus building among communities and nations is an essential foundation for a peaceful and prosperous world. NIGH's goal to inform and empower nurses and others from around the world to become "21st-century Nightingales" is increasing and gaining momentum. To follow more fully in Nightingale's footsteps, we are focused on local and global sustainability strategies for the nursing community. This requires acknowledging the core connections between the integral process, human caring, and human health, as listed in Table 2.1.

NIGH will continue to seek opportunities for collaboration on local and global scales. Through nursing's efforts, doors open, hearts are touched, and families and communities have the potential to be changed for the better. The ongoing sustainability of the NIGH will directly relate to our continuing awareness of the need to be integrally informed and active, as individuals and as a team.

Electronic media will enhance the training of trainer programs, and CD and iPod formats will follow in an effort to inform the world about this journey. Future plans also include the development of related regional and global communities of practice (CoPs) that have already emerged as people seek more ways to become involved and to be supported.

LESSONS LEARNED AND WORDS OF WISDOM

Our efforts have helped us realize that our work embraces feminine principles of leadership. The feminine allows for the creating of a sacred healing presence and space to allow us to acknowledge our shared vision, our shared suffering. By so doing, we can contribute to create optimal healing environments—both internal and external. As this is done, we contribute to the flow of meaning between or among individuals who seek to understand others' points of view related to various aspects of being human from the micro (personal) level to the macro (societal) level. We thus enter into that dialogue process where we come together to share worldview, meaning, feelings, and experiences to establish trust and community in the deepest sense.

As we continue to evolve, learn, and integrate integral principles, practices, theories, and approaches into our own lives, we are experiencing the depth of how each can become a member of a larger "healing community and healing environment." This journey supports us to move with more harmony and balance, and the barriers to our ideals begin to dissolve. We understand that we—as individuals, as a NIGH team, and as a part of our worldwide nursing community—are indeed a few of the vital change agents who can create the cultural shifts needed in our own homes, families, workplaces, and communities. We sense that we can achieve vibrant, vigorous, and healthier healthcare systems worldwide, moving towards that healthier world we envision. Individually, we are each writing our role in history as we commit ourselves anew to improve "self-care" and to nurture the collective networks that can actualize our visions for a healthy world. Collectively, we are humbled to be working with so many people and organizations toward the adoption of the UNRs, as we prepare for the celebration of 2010: International Year of the Nurse, and as we commit to implementing 2011–2020: UN Decade for a Healthy World.

REFERENCES

Buresh, B., and Gordon, S. (2000). *From silence to voice: What nurses know and must communicate to the public.* Ottawa. Canadian Nurses Association.

Dossey, B. M. (in press). Integral and holistic nursing: Local to global. In Dossey, B.M., & Keegan, L. *Holistic Nursing: A Handbook for Practice* (5th ed.). Sudbury, MA: Jones and Bartlett Publishers.

Dossey, B. M. (in press). Theory of Integral Nursing. In Dossey, B.M., & Keegan, L. *Holistic Nursing: A Handbook for Practice* (5th ed.). Sudbury, MA: Jones and Bartlett Publishers.

Dossey, B. M., Selanders, L. C., Beck, D. M., and Attewell, A. (2005). *Florence Nightingale today Healing, leadership, global action.* (pp. 151-171). Washington, DC: NurseBooks.Org.

Halifax. J., Dossey. B. M., & Rushton, C. H. (2007). *Compassionate care of the dying.* (pp. 105–106). Santa Fe, NM: Prajna Mountain Press.

International Council of Nurses (ICN) (2004). The global shortage of registered nurses: An overview of issues and action. Retrieved April 1, 2007, at http://www.icn.ch/global/shortage.pdf

Karpf, T., Tashima, N., & Crain, C. (2008). *Restoring hope: Building a foundation for decent care.* WHO Copenhagen, Denmark, WHO. Nightingale. F. (1860). *Notes on nursing: What it is, and what it is not.* London: Harrison and Sons.

Nightingale, F. (1893). Sick-nursing and health-nursing. In Beck, D. M. (2005). *Sick-nursing and health-nursing: Nightingale establishes our broad scope of practice in 1893.* In Dossey, B. M., Selanders, L. C., Beck, D. M., and Attewell, A. *Florence Nightingale today: Healing, leadership, global action.* (p. 296). Washington, DC: NurseBooks.Org.

Reich, W. T. (1989). Speaking of suffering: A moral account of compassion. *Soundings,* 72:83–108.

United Nations Millennium Development Goals (2000). New York: United Nations. Retrieved April 1, 2007, at http://www.un.org/millenniumgoals/goals.html

Wilber, K. (1999). *The collected works of Ken Wilber* (Vols. 1-4). Boston: Shambhala.

Wilber, K. (2000a). *The collected works of Ken Wilber* (Vols. 5-8). Boston: Shambhala.

Wilber, K. (2000b). *Integral psychology.* Boston: Shambhala.

World Health Organization. (2006). Report of the World Health Organization Forum for Government Chief Nursing and Midwifery Officers. Geneva: WHO.

World Health Organization. (2007). Restoring hope: Building a foundation for decent care. Copenhagen, Denmark (European WHO Office): WHO.

CHAPTER 3

Two to Tango— the Pleasure and Pain of International Collaboration

Jane Salvage, BA, MSc, RGN, HonLLD

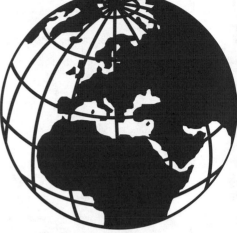

International collaboration between nurses can be useful and rewarding, professionally and personally, for everyone involved. The opportunity to work with, learn from, and develop lasting relationships with nurses from a different country and culture can be one of life's most enriching experiences.

My definition of international collaboration is intentionally wide, covering any activity where nurses from different countries join in partnership with the ultimate goal of improving health and healthcare. This can be as apparently simple as a visit by an expert to another country to share her knowledge or as complex as a major international project with many participating countries and funding sources.

Networking on a regional and even global scale is growing stronger in nursing. More scope for collaboration exists than ever before. Funding is more readily available, while easier travel and instant communication have overcome many barriers to joint work. All too often, however, international collaboration brings few rewards but

much misunderstanding and frustration and wastes time and money. This is especially likely when nurses from a richer, supposedly more developed country work with colleagues from a poorer country in an unequal donor-recipient relationship.

International collaboration to promote sustainable development is never easy. It requires particular skills and strong motivation. However, by following some simple rules based on clear values, nursing projects can achieve great results for all involved. Whatever the type and scale of collaboration, universally relevant underlying themes and principles do exist.

The Context

Globalisation is having an impact on nursing just as it is on most other fields of human endeavour. Nurses are now much more likely to travel to other countries not only for holidays, but also for work, whether to gain experience or money in a different country or to participate in a project. Travel is cheaper and easier than it has ever been. Even those who do not travel or have low incomes have more opportunities than ever before to communicate across national borders via phone, fax, e-mail, or the Internet.

The impact of the explosion in international collaboration can be felt in nursing as in other fields. Books, conferences, journals (electronic as well as paper), videoconferencing, satellite links, e-mail, and the Internet are all channels of communication increasingly used by nurses, and the coming years will bring yet more innovations. They provide a backdrop and stimulus to the many types of collaborative projects in which nurses are involved— whether it is a small-scale twinning project between two colleges of nursing, a bilateral government-funded project to improve primary health care in a developing country, a joint European Masters programme, a multi-centre comparative research study, or a series of multinational meetings to draw up guidelines on mental health care.

Globalisation also provides the backdrop to the growth and development of nursing as an industry. A greater understanding now exists that health problems do not respect national boundaries (the human immunodeficiency virus, tuberculosis, and avian influenza provide obvious examples). Richer countries, now as always, offer help to poorer ones not only for altruistic reasons, but also to exert political influence. As the gap between rich and poor looms as wide as ever, rich governments and international agencies such as the United Nations (UN) are under pressure to soften the harsh impact of free market capitalism through aid programmes of all kinds, as well as through disaster relief. And as billions of dollars pour into projects, the aid field has changed out of recognition—from an amateurish pursuit for high-minded volunteers into a huge, professionalised industry.

Meanwhile nursing participation in international affairs remains relatively marginal, as the profession continues to struggle against the traditional obstacles of lack of power and status that stem from gender discrimination and the medicalisation of healthcare. It is difficult to secure funding for nursing development projects in all parts of the world and difficult to persuade powerful agencies like the World Bank and the World Health Organization (WHO) that nursing is a major contributor to health gain, worthy of as much support as medicine. Nevertheless, slow progress is being made. Access to European Union (EU) funding is one example: As nurses have learned how to work the system, and as they have increased their capacity to conduct research, write proposals, and run good projects, more funding has started to come their way.

All this activity generates new business opportunities and opens up new markets. Nursing colleges are recruiting growing numbers of overseas nurses—not only to fill staff gaps in western countries, but also to provide the higher education for nurses that many countries still lack. The newfound focus on continuing professional development likewise stimulates the production of books, journals, distance learning courses, conferences, and web sites, many of them designed to generate income.

Finally, completing this rapid sketch of some key background factors is the question of language. English is or is becoming the dominant common language in many parts of the world, with the wealth and power of the United States (US) and its global media reinforcing language bias handed down from the United Kingdom's (UK) imperial past. This brings difficulties as well as gains. Not least, nurses who speak English as their mother tongue have an inbuilt advantage in international meetings and projects where it is usually assumed that English is the working language. They have to guard against allowing this accident of birth to lead them to dominate such gatherings and impose their values, cultures, and working systems on others.

The Pleasures

Why do we do it? International collaboration is often, though not always, driven by altruism—the desire to help others without any thought of gain for us. Most of us also do it because we enjoy it. Our enjoyment can take many forms.

Altruism

Doing international work helps us feel we are making a contribution, helping to make a difference. In particular, those of us from richer countries may feel inspired, perhaps obliged, to play our part in making the world a better place by sharing some of the knowledge and experience we have been fortunate to acquire. Nurses in many poor countries have little access to the education, professional development, career opportunities, and rewards that many nurses in richer countries enjoy. The chance to use these advantages to reduce suffering and improve health is a life-enriching privilege.

Fun, Friendship, Excitement

My international work has provided me with some of the most enjoyable and exciting experiences of my life, in personal as well as professional terms. I have made lasting friendships with people all round the world and visited amazing places.

Personal Development

My international work has helped me to grow as a person, to learn more about life, and to question my assumptions about what matters in life, how things should be done, or what the best way is to live.

Professional Development

International collaboration teaches new professional knowledge and skills, as long as the participants approach it with an open mind. It has taught me about many new ways of thinking about health and healthcare and many new practices. It has helped me to develop my skills in facilitation, consultancy, assessment, problem-solving, strategic planning, fundraising, project management, and public speaking. My knowledge of foreign languages has also improved.

Health Gain

This perhaps should be first on the list of pleasures, although too many projects are unable to demonstrate that they lead to any health gain. People from different countries may come together, have a good time, learn a lot, and go home satisfied, but that in itself will not necessarily improve the health of people in their countries. We need to be much more rigorous in focusing on how to achieve better health outcomes through international collaboration.

The Pains

The pleasures are obvious, but what about the pains? Anyone who has worked on an international collaboration has probably experienced some of the following.

Hard Feelings

Feelings like frustration, disappointment, and anger are more common than we would like to admit. People who set out with good intentions may find that nothing goes according to plan. The project partners may be unhappy with the way things are going; communications may be poor, and misunderstandings frequent; and cultural and linguistic differences, often a source of delight, can turn sour and lead to broken promises and unfulfilled commitments. External obstacles such as political complications, even corruption, can poison the best-intentioned activities. The anger, sadness and frustration felt on all sides may be difficult to acknowledge and handle.

Inappropriate Processes, Methods, and Solutions

This is an extremely common failing. Through lack of experience, or feelings of superiority bred by differences of gender, race, profession, culture and history, people often—perhaps even usually—embark on projects without paying enough attention to the processes they use. Skilled facilitation and consensus-building based on an explicit framework of shared values and goals are needed, not as luxuries but as essential ingredients of a successful project. Collaboration often assumes that the technical content is what matters, such as sharing expertise on safe motherhood, but the how of project management is as important as the what. If the how is not properly managed, the what will not take root. And this leads to…

Lack of Sustainability

Many projects, even if they make it to the end, leave little trace behind. Their imprint is washed away by the next tide like footprints in the sand. Like research studies whose results are not disseminated, they may sound impressive but do absolutely nothing to change practice or improve health. No one likes to admit this, and project reports often fail to give an honest account of what happened. Thus, poor concepts or incompetent consultants move from one project to the next. More forethought and honesty could minimise this waste of human effort, money, and potential.

(Nursing) Imperialism

Many of the previously mentioned problems arise from imperialistic or neocolonial attitudes. Although most countries are not colonies any more, the rich and powerful see their development role as teaching less enlightened people to do things their way. Wealth does help to create the conditions for learning to do some things better, but not always and not automatically. Nurses from rich countries, used to being low in the medical or political hierarchy, do not perceive themselves as oppressors, but they can be just as domineering as the old colonial masters, even if they do it in a nicer way. They assume that their ways of seeing, their knowledge, and their systems are the best.

Their partners in poorer countries often fail to challenge them, through politeness, cultural norms, lack of self-confidence, lack of fluency in the project's main language, political pressure, or fear that desperately needed money and support will be withdrawn. I am reminded of the wise words of a German development worker living in Mongolia: "You cannot tell people what to do. You can only help them to do what they want to do. Your task is to help them see what is possible, by talking, asking, demanding reactions and ideas. It has to come from them, from below to above. What do they, the people, want? All you can do is suggest. Then if they agree, you can act."

Towards Some Guidelines

Effective international collaboration is far harder than we like to admit. There is almost a conspiracy of silence about it. But the good news is that it is possible, provided we go about it in the right way. I would like to offer some simple guidelines as a foundation for international collaboration between nurses, based on my own experience and observations and input from colleagues. It may sound like I'm stating the obvious, but these guidelines are so often ignored that they bear repeating. I have evolved them through many mistakes and successes in my 20-odd years of experience as an international health and nursing consultant.

The checklist below offers advice on these points: preparation, sensitivity, language and culture, values and visions, planning, monitoring and evaluation, involving stakeholders, dissemination, and practicalities.

1. Do Your Homework

My involvement in an international project often starts with the atlas and moves on to the guidebook. Unbelievable as it may seem, nurses will get on a plane to another country without even knowing where it is, let alone its recent history, its political system, or what languages are spoken. They waste hours and days of others' time and scarce project resources asking their hosts for information they could have found out before they left home. The Internet leaves no excuses for ignorance, and there are many other good sources of data and networks to provide experienced contacts. So let's do our homework first.

2. Be Sensitive and Imaginative

As you do your homework, you should be alert to issues that may be complex, painful, or culturally difficult to address. The best possible attitude when entering a joint project of any kind is to be open and sensitive, especially if you are the more wealthy, privileged, or powerful partner. Use your imagination to get inside the partner's skin, experiencing and seeing as much of their culture and environment as possible—not just the main hospital or hotel meeting room. Look at how ordinary people live, not only the ministry officials and university lecturers. Remember that your hosts may want to show you the best of what they have, giving you an unbalanced picture of the current situation. When they invite you to their home for a meal, you may unwittingly eat food that the family would normally live on for a week or work for a month to buy.

3. Be Aware of Language and Culture

Good communication is the key factor in creating openness and mutual understanding. Learning a new language for a project may be impractical, but anyone can look at a phrasebook and learn a few greetings, thereby showing respect for the culture and awareness of its language. Don't assume, as so many visitors do, that the locals speak your language, and don't assume that an interpreter will be provided. Discuss this in advance and allocate necessary funds to pay professional interpreters and translators. Be patient and supportive when partners communicate in your language, and speak clearly and simply. The politics of language can be a minefield, so don't take anything for granted. Equally, you may be oblivious to cultural misunderstandings that can undermine relationships, so the more you know about your hosts, the better. Remember, too, that you will be seen as a representative of your country, profession, and institution, so act accordingly.

4. SHARE VALUES AND VISIONS

Every collaboration should start with mutual exploration of dreams and visions. Underlying values and assumptions can be disclosed and debated through open discussion of what everyone hopes to achieve. Formal sessions should be structured for this purpose, in addition to informal social gatherings. You are likely to find many shared values, but also differences, according to culture and individual preference. Exploring them at the beginning of collaboration, as well as later in the process, builds a firm foundation for the work and creates an atmosphere in which difficulties can be resolved earlier and more easily. Otherwise, you might be in for some nasty surprises. Handling diversity needs to be a theme throughout: no one should embark on joint work without considering the impact of the partners' varied backgrounds and assumptions. Divergence of opinion or approach is often feared and covered up, when it can actually be the most creative and inspiring aspect of collaboration.

5. PLAN THE WORK

Some projects develop immensely complicated and elaborate plans before the partners have even met, while others are impossibly vague. You need to steer a middle course, combining clarity and purposefulness with flexibility. Never assume everyone understands what the project is about; spend plenty of time at the beginning working through the plan, ensuring that absolutely everyone who matters is clear about it and agrees with it and that all doubts and fears have been explored. This requires open, participative, democratic discussions led by someone with excellent facilitation skills. The project leader is often too heavily involved to be a good facilitator, and it may be worth considering inviting someone else to do this. Not only will their skills be useful, but also they should be, and should be seen to be, impartial.

6. Monitor and Evaluate

Talk, talk, and more talk is needed, not just at the beginning but throughout. Each step of the project should be monitored, and each next step planned in the light of this evaluation. The tools may be simple and informal, supplementing the more formal evaluation systems and reports most projects require. It is important to document these in writing as project personnel may change and as a record for review later. You must be prepared to make major changes to the project as it develops. Few really creative projects go the way you expect. Most will have surprises, twists and turns, disasters and unexpected successes; you must be open to the outcomes and not force the project down a predetermined path.

7. Involve the Stakeholders

Many a hopeful project has hit the rocks halfway through when it was discovered that another project team was already doing the same work. I remember a bitter experience where two teams of nurse educators from two western countries were busily working with local nurses in a country in eastern Europe on what they thought would be the new national curriculum. The Ministry of Health and the local nurses did not tell either team of the other's existence, leading, when it was discovered, to wasted effort, anger, and no curriculum! It is vital from the beginning to find out who else is active in your area and to design your project to complement or build on previous and ongoing work—or even better, to join forces with the "competition." Creating and maintaining excellent links with senior managers, policymakers, and other stakeholders is vital here. Their support will be essential not only for your project, but also for helping achieve the attitudinal shifts without which no nursing development can be sustained.

8. Disseminate

Once the project is over, it is human nature to move on to the next activity without harvesting what was learned. Many international projects are required to produce a final report for donors, but these are too rarely turned into articles for publication that could guide and inspire others. Conference presentations and journal articles that spell out the outcomes, achievements, and lessons learned are developmental for the project partners, useful for seeking future support, a boost for morale, and sometimes inspirational for others.

9. REMEMBER THE PRACTICALITIES

Finally, many people travel overseas to visit project partners with little thought for the practicalities involved. Travel and health insurance, visas and invitation letters, preventive health measures before and during your visit, communication home via phone and e-mail, and knowing what to do in an emergency should all be considered in advance. You should be in good health and well informed on how to stay healthy in the country you are visiting, including coping with jet lag, a different diet, and a different climate. Be aware, too, of the power of "culture shock," a natural experience for all travelers. Without your even knowing, it can generate deep-seated anxieties that affect your emotions and the clarity you need to work well. Homesickness, lack of direction, insomnia, mood swings, loss of confidence, fatigue, and illness cannot be ruled out, but you can take steps to keep them to a minimum.

COLLABORATIVE SUCCESSES: TWO EXAMPLES

A wealth of success stories in international collaboration between nurses exist. I'd like to mention two from my time working with WHO that gave me particular satisfaction.

NATIONAL ACTION PLANS FOR ESTONIA AND FINLAND

Nurse leaders in the newly independent ex-Soviet republic of Estonia wanted to develop a new vision and direction for nursing, which had been neglected and undervalued for many years. They asked me, in my former role as WHO regional nursing adviser for Europe, for help. After discussions we decided to hold a workshop to bring together 20 or so key figures in the Estonian nursing world and develop a national action plan. Nurses from Finland, a neighbouring country that was building closer links with Estonia, responded warmly to our request for assistance, and we jointly facilitated a 3-day workshop in Estonia, which produced a strategy and much enthusiasm. The Finnish nurses secured funding from their government and employers and continued to support the Estonians over the coming years— with both sides describing it as an important learning experience. For example, the Finnish nurses realised that they themselves did not have an adequate action plan for nursing, so they started work on one; the most recent version was presented to the Finnish parliament in 2004.

LEARNING MATERIALS FOR EASTERN EUROPE

In the early 1990s, nurses from the countries of Central and Eastern Europe (CEE) and the former Soviet Union (NIS) were beginning to make contact with others and to work on plans for reform. But most lacked textbooks or journals in their own language, making progress almost impossible. Therefore, my WHO colleague Adele Beerling and I launched a project to produce a basic nursing manual that would bridge the gap until countries could generate their own literature. It was called the Learning Materials on Nursing (LEMON). We brought together experts from east and west, who attended many meetings and put in many hours of unpaid work. Together we compiled a package of learning materials that was, as far as possible, culturally neutral and based on universal nursing principles. This was adapted and translated into many different languages and is still being used by thousands of practitioners and teachers in Bosnia and Herzegovina, Croatia, the Czech Republic, Estonia, Hungary, Kyrgyzstan, Latvia, Romania, Russia, Slovakia, Slovenia, Tajikistan, Uzbekistan, and elsewhere. Nurses in all these countries persuaded a range of donors to fund some of the work and raised local stakeholders' awareness of nursing issues.

CONCLUSION

Much more professionalism is needed if we are to develop sustainable, effective projects that can also give donors proof of the value of investing in nursing. These simple beginnings of a set of guidelines for international project work may help. They are actually principles we use, or should use, in any project, whether it is international or not. Similar principles underlie the provision of good patient care. Some of them can be found in the literature on project management and on development.

Nurses involved in international work should be aware of and work in the broader discipline of international development studies, so they can learn from others but also make their own distinctive contribution. Nursing projects often go forward in isolation from the mainstream, but we have much to learn from the international experience of experts in other disciplines, and something of our own to contribute. Those involved in international collaboration should see themselves not only as nurses, but also as development professionals.

It is a cliché in international circles to say that we learn much from our own and others' experiences, but like most clichés it is true. We learn only if we are open to learning, however, and open to the discomfort and challenge that can involve. Too often the learning is one-way, if there is any learning at all—the rich assuming they are teaching the poor and paying lip service to the idea that they can learn from the poor in their turn. It really does take two to tango, and if you enter the work with an open heart and a mind ready to question and explore, you will reap wonderful professional, intellectual, and personal rewards.

This paper has evolved through various drafts and commentaries, starting with a presentation given at the International Council of Nurses congress, Copenhagen, Denmark, June 12, 2001, and a posting on the *Nursing Times* web site, http://www.nursingtimes.net, July 26, 2001. Special thanks to Doris Christensen, Betty Kershaw, Robert Pratt, and Karenlene Ravn for their valuable insights. Comments, criticisms, and additions, including information about any existing guidelines that might be utilized, are warmly welcomed. Send e-mail to work@janesalvage.me.uk.

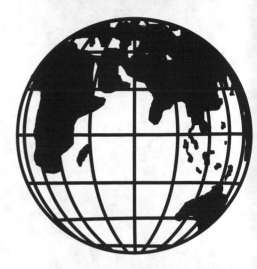

PART II

WISDOM

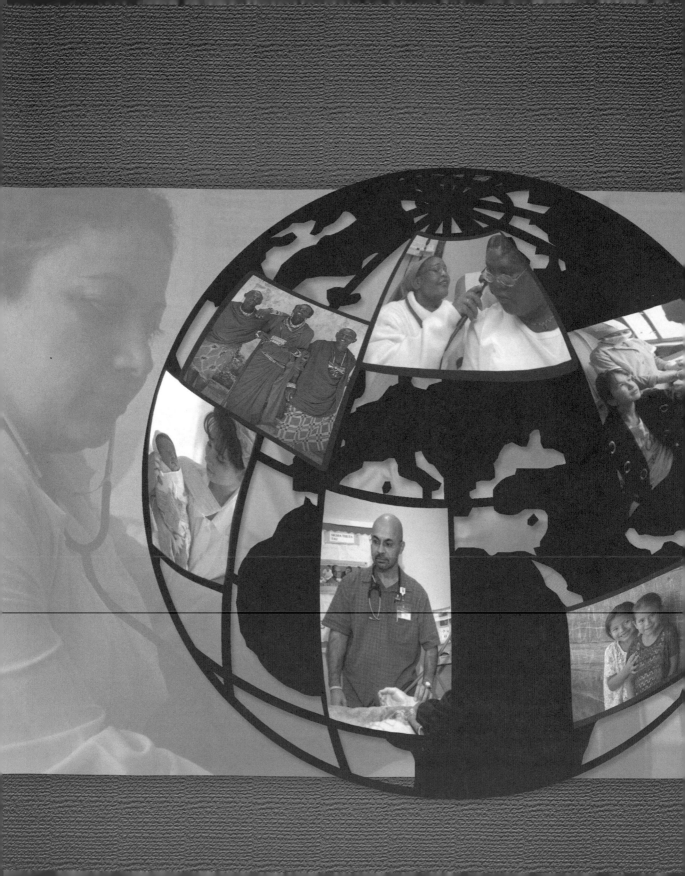

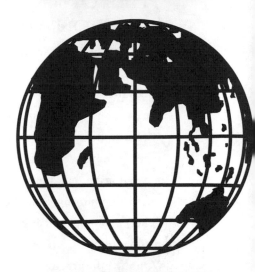

THE INTERNATIONAL NURSING LEADERSHIP INSTITUTE (INLI)

SHARON M. WEINSTEIN, MS, RN, CRNI, FAAN
ELENA STEMPOVSCAIA, PhD, RN
K. JANE YOUNGER, MSN, RN

With the dissolution of the former Soviet Union in the 1990s, a plethora of new independent states evolved, and at the same time, something ended. Members of the healthcare community, once linked by a common country, were no longer able to communicate with their former colleagues through international conferences and symposia.

Early in 1992, nursing emerged as a key issue throughout the new independent states of the former Soviet Union (NIS) and Central and Eastern European (CEE) countries. Cognizant of the need to tackle nursing issues within the context of a partnership model, United States (US) nurse leaders developed Nursing Task Forces to meet the challenges of nurses at an institutional level and to provide a forum for the exchange of ideas and lessons learned. The Task Forces were the driving force behind the nursing agenda with a focus on three areas: education, practice, and leadership.

CHAPTER 4

THE POWER OF PARTNER-TO-PARTNER RELATIONSHIPS

The American International Health Alliance (AIHA), founded in 1992 through a cooperative agreement with the United States Agency for International Development (USAID), facilitated communications and partnerships between U.S. healthcare providers and their foreign counterparts, but more importantly, across country lines. Nurses, previously considered mid-level personnel, have benefited from these changes more than any other group by becoming part of an ongoing community of nurse leaders and scholars. Initial efforts by U.S. nurse partners focused on relationship building—relationships between U.S. and foreign hospitals and between U.S. and foreign nursing leaders. Colleagues worked diligently to build a base of knowledge related to clinical practice, a nursing curriculum, and nursing associations. The programs flourished, and a nursing infrastructure was created in countries throughout the former NIS and CEE countries. With the infrastructure came a base from which to value nursing's past and create nursing's future. Hundreds of nurses participated in exchange programs to and from the US and the new countries. Annual conferences were held to unite the U.S. partners with their new counterparts and to unite nurse leaders from throughout the NIS/CEE countries with their counterparts. Nurses from Armenia were now in dialogue with nurses from Russia and Albania. Nurses from Moldova had Internet access and communication with their counterparts from Turkmenistan.

THE EVOLUTION OF THE INTERNATIONAL NURSING LEADERSHIP INSTITUTE

Building on the success of these programs, Dr. Weinstein and her colleagues created the International Nursing Leadership Institute (INLI), a unique year-long, three-session, learning experience designed for nurse leaders in collaborative practice partnerships.

Using adult learning principles and an interactive approach to learning resulted in the creation of a cadre of developing leaders for developing nations. The strategy could be implemented in any emerging country, but was targeted to the NIS/CEE countries. Nurses in the NIS and CEE faced numerous challenges following the dissolution of the former Soviet Union (Table 4.1). Unlike their colleagues in the United States and western Europe, the role of the nurses in these regions was viewed as an extension of the physician's role—as a mid-level worker rather than as an independent professional. Lack of professional standards, the absence of nurses in positions of power and influence, low status, insufficient pay, high turnover, and low morale—all presented an opportunity for significant change. Thus, the partnership model evolved, creating the first nursing initiative in 1992 (Weinstein & Brooks, 2003).

TABLE 4.1.   PARTICIPANT COUNTRIES: INLI PROGRAM.

New Independent States	Central/Eastern Europe
Russian Federation	Albania
Caucuses	Croatia
Armenia	Latvia
Azerbaijan	Romania
Georgia	
Central Asian Republics	
Kazakhstan	
Kyrgyzstan	
Tajikistan	
Turkmenistan	
Uzbekistan	
West NIS	
Belarus	
Moldova	
Ukraine	

QUALITY MANAGEMENT OUTCOMES AND SUSTAINABILITY

Significant outcomes evolved as a result of this program.

EDUCATION

A series of conferences in-country focused on education and curriculum reforms. Local Nursing Resource Centers (NRCs) provided nursing faculty, students, and practitioners with alternative forms of learning. Each site was equipped with computers, textbooks, videotapes, anatomical models, and educational posters addressing clinical, managerial, and psychosocial aspects of healthcare. The Centers have encouraged independent learning and enhanced traditional teaching methodologies. Nurses attest to the impact of the nursing initiative and the NRCs on their profession.

Basic nursing education in the NIS/CEE has traditionally been viewed as vocational training, rather than university-based. With a faculty comprised primarily of physician nurse educators, a move toward development of a cadre of nurse faculty evolved. The natural starting point was the creation of a baccalaureate-level model. Traditionally, baccalaureate and advanced practice nursing were not available in all countries. Nursing education has now expanded from a 2-year program to advanced clinical and management training. Four-year baccalaureate nursing programs and continuous learning have become commonplace; such programs include skills laboratories, postgraduate training, and the extensive use of the NRCs.

International nursing conferences have extended the learning process, and NIS/CEE nurses have attended the International Council of Nurses (ICN) meetings in London and Copenhagen. Truly, second-generation leaders have evolved.

Clinical Practice

Changes in clinical practice occurred with the introduction of clinical practice guidelines, nursing standards, policies, and procedures. Process workshops introduced practice patterns that have transformed nursing's role and image. Countries such as Kyrgyzstan and Russia have seen the development of new nursing roles for clinical nurse educators, clinical managers, and nurse teachers.

Leadership

The first nursing association in Russia was founded in 1992 as a voice for the nursing profession before the government, other non-governmental organizations, and the public at large. Although delegates from 44 regions of the Russian Federation emerged as fledgling leaders, they lacked the experience and advocacy skills necessary to enter into a policy dialogue with local officials. Training in organizational development and strategy formulation to influence policy change supportive of the nursing profession contributed to the success of these associations, which now exist in all countries of the former NIS/CEE. The All Russian Nursing Association, which follows the federation model, has been accepted for membership in the ICN.

CHALLENGES

In creating the model NRC, we underestimated physician interest in the materials, space, and access. We should have partnered with physicians as appropriate to involve them in the educational process. Because many of them felt deprived from both the learning and travel experiences, they took control of the resource materials and centers in some of the Central Asian Republics, arguing that physicians, by virtue of their education, should have access to more than nurses did.

LESSONS LEARNED

Leaders have historically helped others to integrate their personal values with the values of the workplace—and helped to explain the paradoxes when values collided. Because senior nurses in the NIS/CEE countries have always taken a back seat to physician administrators within their respective institutions, it was essential that they develop the skills associated with senior leadership roles. Many participants in the first INLI class had traveled to the US and had seen their counterparts in the work environments in which they practiced. The partnership model set the stage for development and helped to identify emerging nurse leaders in each country and in each region. Over a 3-year period, these early leaders became presidents and executive directors of local nursing associations and chief nurses of their respective health ministries. The INLI format satisfied the next phase of the leadership model—the ability to sustain the successes and disseminate them to a larger pool of nurses.

Our goal was to create a cadre of nurse leaders/educators. Initial faculty were chosen from U.S. nurse leaders with experience in the NIS/CEE countries. We used adult learning methods to create an integrated curriculum, graduating the learner into an ongoing community of colleagues and peers. The learners responded well to the mentoring and co-teaching experience, and they were eventually able to replace U.S. nurse faculty. Instruction was active, student-centered, and based on the learner's goals. We created an environment that had "real-life" application for the material being learned, that built on previous life experiences, and that promoted positive self-esteem and self-worth (Training Post, 2003). Faculty used a series of leading management books to generate the curriculum (see Box 4.1). Students and faculty, in full costume, acted out the stories. For example, the parable *Who Moved My Cheese* (Johnson, 1998) encouraged students to have contingency plans and to expect change. A maze was created, and students moved through the maze to reach their destinations, facing multiple stumbling blocks along the way, including a shortage of cheese (supplies). The book *The Oz Principle* (Connors, Smith, & Hickman, 1998) told students that they could be or do whatever they wanted…if they wanted it badly enough! The author contended that like Dorothy and her companions in *The Wizard of Oz*, most people in the corporate world possess the power within themselves to get the results they need. Instead, they behave as though they were victims of circumstance. The authors demonstrated how anyone can move beyond making excuses to obtain the results they want, an important leadership tool. Faculty became the characters and led the students through the story, ending in Dorothy's ability to return home as a result of the power within her. The book *Goldilocks on Management* (Mayer & Mayer, 1999) featured a series of revisionist fairy tales for serious managers. A message from the author's story of *Chicken Little* reminded students that they could control rumors with timely, accurate, and effective communication. Costumes, props, and teamwork enriched the course content.

Critical thinking is an imperative for the professional nurse. A number of quantitative researchers have studied and measured the associated skills for critical thinking (Weinstein, 2005; Andrews, 1999). The Neuman Systems Model was used to explore its application to foreign nurse leaders by building on the concept of intervention to strengthen the line of defense for or deal with interpersonal and extrapersonal environmental stressors. To gain these skill sets and apply interventions, INLI students participated in thought-provoking exercises in the classroom, worked collaboratively in small cross-country groups, and completed reflection journal entries. Students were also required to develop a project with local ministry and institutional approval. Assignments and presentations were critiqued for evidence of critical thinking, such as identifying, defining, collaborating, prioritizing, choosing options, clarifying, and summarizing.

Lessons on systems enabled the learner to understand "big picture thinking" and the impact of change in complex systems. Once we embrace the idea that systems thinking can improve individual learning by inducing people to focus on the whole system, and by providing individuals with the skills and tools to enable them to derive observable patterns of behavior from the systems they see at work, the next step is to justify why this process is so important to organizations of people (Porter-O'Grady, 2005).

BOX 4.1.   CORE SUBJECTS COVERED IN THE YEAR-LONG INLI CURRICULUM.

SESSION ONE

Leadership competencies

Adult learning principles

Expectations of INLI participants/faculty

Group norms and group dynamics

Introduction of the theme

Project development, management, and monitoring

Computer skills

Teamwork

Publishing/dissemination strategies

Communicating with diverse audiences

Evaluation methodologies

SESSION TWO

SWOT analysis

Time, change, and barrier management

Performance appraisals/human resource management

Systems thinking

Continuous quality improvement

Meeting planning

Influencing policy development

Negotiation/conflict resolution

SESSION THREE

Ethics

Critical thinking

Customer service

Professional development

Mentoring and coaching

Developing strategic partnerships

Lessons on the use of "cause and effect thinking" helped students to understand organizational issues. Participants learned about 360-degree performance appraisals and the importance of feedback from multiple sources. Guest faculty from global nursing organizations such as Sigma Theta Tau International Honor Society (STTI), the American Organization of Nurse Executives (AONE), the World Health Organization (WHO), and the International Council of Nurses (ICN) enhanced the quality of the education. For example, Patricia Thompson (STTI) taught the students a Scholarly Approach to Leadership, and Kirsten Stallkneckt (ICN) addressed the students on the ICN mission and her role as president.

Based on faculty input, classroom content, and project development, participants were asked to rate the teaching team's effectiveness in using resources, time, materials, group activities, and interpreters. Post graduation, participants were encouraged to continue to work with INLI graduates in their respective countries of the NIS and CEE. Armed with the talent and tools needed to advance in their respective nursing careers, the first class graduated in June, 2000. Four graduates were selected to serve as faculty for the next round of training workshops. Subsequent classes achieved similar results, and 34 of the 60 graduates have been granted international membership in AONE and/or have been inducted as community leaders in STTI.

SUSTAINED NURSING LEADERSHIP—THE FUTURE

INLI has served as the primary vehicle for the development of sustained nursing leadership for the region. A competitive fellowship program for INLI graduates awarded small project grants to nurses from NIS/CEE countries. This seed money has facilitated growth and the ability to complete INLI projects locally. As a result of the partner-to-partner program and participation in INLI, former staff nurses and nurse managers have achieved recognition as presidents of local and national nursing associations, as faculty in colleges and schools of nursing, and as ministry chief nurses. The partnership model has empowered them to be more resourceful and independent; to be critical thinkers; to plan for nursing's future; to educate colleagues, patients, and the community; to manage departments, nursing units, and organizations; to represent their organization and profession to the public; and to speak with one collective voice. In short, they are second-generation leaders.

Through the exceptional leadership of nurse leaders, nurse educators, and clinicians in the developing nations of the NIS and CEE, the discipline and practice of nursing has advanced in a multitude of ways that serve the people from all regions and have produced cross-country linkages. INLI served as the foundation…the future remains to unfold.

REFERENCES

Andrews, M. (1999). *Transcultural concepts in nursing care* (3rd Ed.). (p. 535). Philadelphia: Lippincott Williams & Williams.

Connors, R., Smith, T., & Hickman, C.R. (1998). *The Oz principle.* (pp. 57, 169). Paramus: Prentice Hall.

Johnson, S. (1998). *Who moved my cheese?* (pp. 44–61). New York: G.P. Putnam.

Mayer, G.G. & Mayer T. (1999). *Goldilocks on management.* (pp.123-132). New York: Amacom (American Management Association).

Porter-O'Grady, T. (2005). Critical thinking for nurse leadership. *Nurse Leader*, 3(4).

Training Post (2003). How to apply adult learning principles. Retrieved November 20, 2003, from The Training Post: http://www.trainingpost.org/alpover

Weinstein, S. (2005). Nursing leadership. In Feldman, H. & Greenberg, J., *Educating nurses for leadership*. NY: Springer Publishing.

Weinstein, S. & Brooks, A. M. (2003). *Nursing in the NIS/CEE region: changing face.* Reflections on Nursing Leadership, Fourth Quarter, pp. 16–19 and 44.

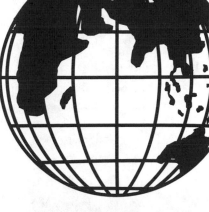

CHAPTER 5

DEVELOPING STANDARDS FOR HEALTHY WORK ENVIRONMENTS

RAMÓN LAVANDERO, RN, MA, MSN, FAAN

The phrase "healthy work environment" (HWE) generally evokes the notion of safe physical environments. In America, numerous federal, state, local, and independent agencies and organizations have issued standards to ensure the physical safety in the workplace. However, healthy work environments require more than physical safety to address behaviors that, while often discounted, are known to contribute to unsafe conditions and impede providing safe and appropriate care to patients and families.

Assumed by many to be "soft" issues, those behaviors that involve relationships are considered to be the key to turning around the epidemic of medical errors in American hospitals and its deleterious impact on their financial health (American Association of Critical-Care Nurses, 2005b). The [United States] Institute of Medicine (IOM) further reports that diminished safety and quality in large part exist because dysfunctional systems in American healthcare today inadequately prepare and support the work of otherwise dedicated professionals (Institute of Medicine, 2001).

Compelling evidence supporting the need for standards that address work environment factors beyond physical safety comes from The Joint Commission, formerly Joint Commission on Accreditation of Healthcare Organizations. The commission maintains an extensive statistical database of sentinel events and associated root causes. Sentinel events require immediate investigation and response because they represent "an unexpected occurrence involving death or serious physical or psychological injury, or the risk thereof. Serious injury specifically includes loss of limb or function" (The Joint Commission, 2007a). Aggregate data from 1995–2005 points to communication as the root cause of nearly two in three (65%) sentinel events (The Joint Commission, 2007b).

VitalSmarts, an organizational performance consultancy and source of the best-selling books *Crucial Conversations: Tools for Talking When the Stakes Are High* (Patterson et al., 2002) and *Crucial Confrontations: Tools for Resolving Broken Promises, Violated Expectations, and Bad Behavior* (Patterson et al., 2004), partnered with the American Association of Critical-Care Nurses (AACN) to study how often healthcare professionals witness colleagues breaking rules, making mistakes, failing to offer support, or appearing critically incompetent, yet fail to speak up. Titled *Silence Kills*, survey and interview data from 1,700 nurses, physicians, administrators, and other clinicians found that fewer than one in 10 said anything about what they had seen (Maxfield et al., 2005). The study also found that those who were "confident in their ability to raise these crucial concerns observe better patient outcomes, work harder, are more satisfied, and are more committed to staying in their jobs" (Maxfield et al., 2005).

DEVELOPING AND DISSEMINATING THE HWE STANDARDS

In 2004, AACN made a strategic decision to speak out loudly and boldly by developing national standards for healthy work environments to directly address the vexing behaviors. The evidence had identified a systemic problem reaching well beyond high acuity and critical-care nursing, even beyond the nursing profession itself.

Nevertheless, AACN's leadership understood the association's obligation to honor what has been termed the "pain-directed" ethic. As defined by David Thomas in the *Ethics of Choice* Training Program, the pain-directed ethic states that:

...it is ethical to work first on the issue causing the organization (or your part of it) the most pain, and then to work on the next most painful issue, and so on, in this way creating improvements in the sequence most likely to ensure not only survival but organizational health and prosperity as well. (Thomas, 2003)

Thomas further asserts that "it is unethical to ignore painful issues. By ignoring painful issues, they are allowed to compound, threatening all the more the ability of the organization to accomplish its purpose" (Thomas, 2003).

A nine-person panel reviewed extensive published and unpublished reports to identify six essential standards and critical elements required for their successful implementation. Fifty experts, representing a wide range of roles, high acuity and critical-care settings, and geographic locations where nursing care is provided across the United States (US), validated the standards, critical elements, and explanatory text (AACN, 2005a–b).

The six HWE standards are as follows:

1. *Skilled Communication:* Nurses must be as proficient in communication skills as they are in clinical skills.

2. *True Collaboration:* Nurses must be relentless in pursuing and fostering true collaboration.

3. *Effective Decision Making:* Nurses must be valued and committed partners in making policy, directing and evaluating clinical care, and leading organizational operations.

4. *Appropriate Staffing:* Staffing must ensure the effective match between patient needs and nurse competencies.

5. *Meaningful Recognition:* Nurses must be recognized and must recognize others for the value each brings to the work of the organization.

6. *Authentic Leadership:* Nurse leaders must fully embrace the imperative of a healthy work environment, authentically live it, and engage others in its achievement.

As shown in Figure 5.1, the standards are considered interdependent among each other and with clinical excellence and optimal patient outcomes. The critical elements associated with each standard may be found at the end of this chapter in the section called "American Association of Critical-Care Nurses: Standards for Establishing and Sustaining Healthy Work Environments."

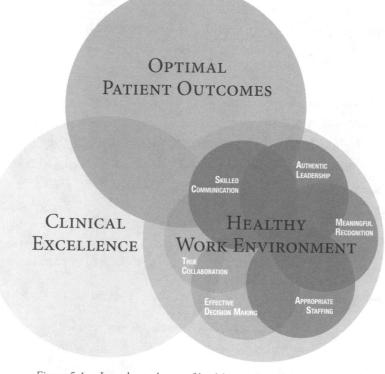

Figure 5.1.   Interdependence of healthy work environment, clinical excellence, and optimal patient outcomes.

Copyright© 2005, American Association of Critical-Care Nurses. Reprinted with permission.

The standards align with the nine provisions of the American Nurses Association Code of Ethics and present a framework by which nurses can practice in conformity with appropriate ethical behavior (American Nurses Association, 2001).

RELEASE AND DISSEMINATION

AACN released the *AACN Standards for Establishing and Sustaining Healthy Work Environments: A Journey to Excellence* in January 2005 at a Washington, DC, press conference along with the compelling results of the *Silence Kills* study (AACN, 2005a–b). Dr. Dennis O'Leary, then president of the Joint Commission, introduced the conference, supporting the need for the standards because of the impact of dysfunctional work environments on patient safety and provider effectiveness.

The standards were announced in widely disseminated news releases. A year-long series presented with Joint Commission Resources, the commission's official publishing and education arm, dedicated an audio conference to each standard. To facilitate maximal access, full text of the standards document including explanatory text, references, and a wide range of additional resources was available for download at no cost from http://www.aacn.org/hwe. Concurrently, communication skill development web seminars (webinars) and workshops were presented in collaboration with VitalSmarts as development of additional assessment and training tools with other partners began.

PROJECT OUTCOMES

During the 2 years since the 2005 press conference when the HWE standards were jointly released with findings from the *Silence Kills* study, 550 media stories were generated. More than 78,000 unique visitors accessed special web sites, downloading more than 135,000 documents, including full text of the standards plus executive summaries of the standards and study findings. More than 1,200 viewers registered for live web seminars on healthy work environments and skilled communication presented through a continuing collaboration between AACN and Vital-Smarts (http://www.vitalsmarts.com). The standards and associated skills training continue to be the subject of countless presentations and workshops at local, regional, and national levels.

Fifteen published articles in leading journals, with another seven under development, are addressing communication, collaboration, leadership, nurse recruitment, and other factors as they relate to healthy work environments (McCauley & Irwin, 2006a; McCauley & Irwin, 2006b; McCauley et al., 2007; Shirey, 2006; Triola, 2006; Hart et al., 2007).

As a baseline for evaluating the impact the impact of standards implementation, AACN, Gannett Healthcare Group, and Bernard Hodes Group, a recruitment and retention consulting division of Omnicom, conducted a national status survey of 4,034 critical-care nurses in the US (Ulrich et al., 2006). When comparing nurses in units and organizations nationally designated or pursuing designation for excellence, this survey also confirmed the intuitive belief that "the pursuit and achievement of excellence does make a difference in how nurses perceive the health of their work environments and nurses' satisfaction with their profession and work compared with other nurses" (Ulrich et al., 2007).

Opportunities, Challenges, and Lessons Learned

The HWE initiative revealed both challenges and opportunities for AACN and for individuals and organizations influenced by the standards. Often, opportunities lay behind each challenge.

Individuals drawn to high acuity and critical-care nursing are generally oriented to immediate action. Not surprisingly, no sooner had the standards been released than committed and concerned professionals began clamoring for assessment tools, implementation guides, and examples of best practices. This posed a time-sensitive challenge, but also opened the opportunity for AACN engage end-user experts and external partners to collaborate in developing resources. The request for examples of best practices generated anecdotal reports and also an article based on the experience of Clarian Health Partners, a three-campus tertiary health system in Indianapolis, Indiana (Kerfoot et al., 2005).

International Interest

Increasing awareness and interest in the standards by countries outside of the US represent both challenge and opportunity. It represents challenge because the standards were developed for American use based on evidence from the American experience. Applicability of the standards for other countries and cultures has not been established, so it cannot be assumed that what works in the US will apply to other countries.

Linguistic translation alone poses unique challenges and should always include so-called back translation. Back translation is "the process of translating a document that has already been translated into a foreign language back into the original language preferably by an independent translator" (Back translation, 2007). Comparing the original and back-translated documents increases the translated document's validity and reliability.

Interest in the standards outside of the US also represents opportunity since expanded implementation offers a unique occasion in which to systematically evaluate whether the HWE standards represent universal elements of healthcare workplaces. AACN has requested that experience and evidence derived from implementation of the standards in other countries and cultures be communicated in writing to the association.

LOOKING AHEAD

The HWE standards were framed for nurses by a professional nursing society, albeit the largest such specialty nursing society in the world. Their applicability beyond nursing, high acuity and critical-care nursing at that, remains to be tested. However, experience since the standards were released confirms their intuitive evidence-based universality. This positions them as a natural rallying point for health professionals and organizations committed to ensuring safety and optimal care for patients and families in every setting.

To date, the American College of Chest Physicians, American Nephrology Nurses Association, American Nurses Association, American Thoracic Society, Association of Nurses in AIDS Care, Emergency Nurses Association, Society of Critical Care Medicine, and the Society of Hospital Medicine have endorsed the standards, with numerous other organizations considering the same.

It remains for the concepts presented in the HWE standards to become fully incorporated into interdisciplinary professional education. This will further cement the IOM call for integrated health professions education as a bridge to quality (Greiner et al., 2003).

Enthusiastic acceptance suggests that the standards resonate at a primal level by giving shape and direction to a perspective sought by many in healthcare. Presentations and published reports will provide evidence of end-user experiences with standards integration. This evidence will inform the next wave of initiatives to assure that successful healthy work environments are sustained.

> *It is ethical to be open to the possibility that your view is incomplete and therefore capable of revision. It is unethical to ignore information that could allow you and/or your organization to grow.*
>
> —David Thomas (2003)

AMERICAN ASSOCIATION OF CRITICAL-CARE NURSES STANDARDS FOR ESTABLISHING AND SUSTAINING HEALTHY WORK ENVIRONMENTS

STANDARD 1—SKILLED COMMUNICATION

Nurses must be as proficient in communication skills as they are in clinical skills.

CRITICAL ELEMENTS

- The healthcare organization provides team members with support for and access to education programs that develop critical communication skills including self-awareness, inquiry/dialogue, conflict management, negotiation, advocacy, and listening.

- Skilled communicators focus on finding solutions and achieving desirable outcomes.

- Skilled communicators seek to protect and advance collaborative relationships among colleagues.

- Skilled communicators invite and hear all relevant perspectives.

- Skilled communicators call upon goodwill and mutual respect to build consensus and arrive at common understanding.

- Skilled communicators demonstrate congruence between words and actions, holding others accountable for doing the same.

- The healthcare organization establishes zero-tolerance policies and enforces them to address and eliminate abuse and disrespectful behavior in the workplace.

- The healthcare organization establishes formal structures and processes that ensure effective information sharing among patients, families, and the healthcare team.

- Skilled communicators have access to appropriate communication technologies and are proficient in their use.

- The healthcare organization establishes systems that require individuals and teams to formally evaluate the impact of communication on clinical, financial, and work environment outcomes.

- The healthcare organization includes communication as a criterion in its formal performance appraisal system and team members demonstrate skilled communication to qualify for professional advancement.

Standard 2—True Collaboration

Nurses must be relentless in pursuing and fostering true collaboration.

Critical Elements

- The healthcare organization provides team members with support for and access to education programs that develop collaboration skills.

- The healthcare organization creates, uses, and evaluates processes that define each team member's accountability for collaboration and how unwillingness to collaborate will be addressed.

- The healthcare organization creates, uses, and evaluates operational structures that ensure the decision making authority of nurses is acknowledged and incorporated as the norm.

- The healthcare organization ensures unrestricted access to structured forums, such as ethics committees, and makes available the time needed to resolve disputes among all critical participants, including patients, families, and the healthcare team.

- Every team member embraces true collaboration as an ongoing process and invests in its development to ensure a sustained culture of collaboration.

- Every team member contributes to the achievement of common goals by giving power and respect to each person's voice, integrating individual differences, resolving competing interests, and safeguarding the essential contribution each must make to achieve optimal outcomes.

- Every team member acts with a high level of personal integrity.

- Team members master skilled communication, an essential element of true collaboration.

- Team member demonstrate competence appropriate to their roles and responsibilities.

- Nurse managers and medical directors are equal partners in modeling and fostering true collaboration.

STANDARD 3—EFFECTIVE DECISION MAKING

Nurses must be valued and committed partners in making policy, directing and evaluating clinical care, and leading organizational operations.

CRITICAL ELEMENTS

- The healthcare organization provides team members with support for and access to ongoing education and development programs focusing on strategies that assure collaborative decision making. Program content includes mutual goal setting, negotiation, facilitation, conflict management, systems thinking, and performance improvement.

- The healthcare organization clearly articulates organizational values, and team members incorporate these values when making decisions.

- The healthcare organization has operational structures in place that ensure the perspectives of patients and their families are incorporated into every decision affecting patient care.

- Individual team members share accountability for effective decision making by acquiring necessary skills, mastering relevant content, assessing situations accurately, sharing fact-based information, communicating professional opinions clearly, and inquiring actively.

- The healthcare organization establishes systems, such as structured forums involving all departments and healthcare disciplines, to facilitate data-driven decisions.

- The healthcare organization establishes deliberate decision making processes that ensure respect for the rights of every individual, incorporate all key perspectives, and designate clear accountability.

- The healthcare organization has fair and effective processes in place at all levels to objectively evaluate the results of decisions, including delayed decisions and indecision.

STANDARD 4—APPROPRIATE STAFFING

Staffing must ensure the effective match between patient needs and nurse competencies.

CRITICAL ELEMENTS

- The healthcare organization has staffing policies in place that are solidly grounded in ethical principles and support the professional obligation of nurses to provide high quality care.

- Nurses participate in all organizational phases of the staffing process from education and planning—including matching nurses' competencies with patients' assessed needs—through evaluation.

- The healthcare organization has formal processes in place to evaluate the effect of staffing decisions on patient and system outcomes. This evaluation includes analysis of when patient needs and nurse competencies are mismatched and how often contingency plans are implemented.

- The healthcare organization has a system in place that facilitates team members' use of staffing and outcomes data to develop more effective staffing models.

- The healthcare organization provides support services at every level of activity to ensure nurses can optimally focus on the priorities and requirements of patient and family care.

- The healthcare organization adopts technologies that increase the effectiveness of nursing care delivery. Nurses are engaged in the selection, adaptation, and evaluation of these technologies.

STANDARD 5—MEANINGFUL RECOGNITION

Nurses must be recognized and must recognize others for the value each brings to the work of the organization.

CRITICAL ELEMENTS

- The healthcare organization has a comprehensive system in place that includes formal processes and structured forums that ensure a sustainable focus on recognizing all team members for their contributions and the value they bring to the work of the organization.

- The healthcare organization establishes a systematic process for all team members to learn about the institution's recognition system and how to participate by recognizing the contributions of colleagues and the value they bring to the organization.

- The healthcare organization's recognition system reaches from the bedside to the board table, ensuring individuals receive recognition consistent with their personal definition of meaning, fulfillment, development, and advancement at every stage of their professional career.

- The healthcare organization's recognition system includes processes that validate that recognition is meaningful to those being acknowledged.

- Team members understand that everyone is responsible for playing an active role in the organization's recognition program and meaningfully recognizing contributions.

- The healthcare organization regularly and comprehensively evaluates its recognition system, ensuring effective programs that help to move the organization toward a sustainable culture of excellence that values meaningful recognition.

STANDARD 6—AUTHENTIC LEADERSHIP

Nurse leaders must fully embrace the imperative of a healthy work environment, authentically live it, and engage others in its achievement.

CRITICAL ELEMENTS

- The healthcare organization provides support for and access to educational programs to ensure that nurse leaders develop and enhance knowledge and abilities in skilled communication, effective decision making, true collaboration, meaningful recognition, and ensuring resources to achieve appropriate staffing.

- Nurse leaders demonstrate an understanding of the requirements and dynamics at the point of care and within this context successfully translate the vision of a healthy work environment.

- Nurse leaders excel at generating visible enthusiasm for achieving the standards that create and sustain healthy work environments.

- Nurse leaders lead the design of systems necessary to effectively implement and sustain standards for healthy work environments.

- The healthcare organization ensures that nurse leaders are appropriately positioned in their pivotal role in creating and sustaining healthy work environments. This includes participation in key decision making forums, access to essential information, and the authority to make necessary decisions.

- The healthcare organization facilitates the efforts of nurse leaders to create and sustain a healthy work environment by providing the necessary time and financial and human resources.

- The healthcare organization provides a formal co-mentoring program for all nurse leaders. Nurse leaders actively engage in the co-mentoring program.

- Nurse leaders role model skilled communication, true collaboration, effective decision making, meaningful recognition, and authentic leadership.

- The healthcare organization includes the leadership contribution to creating and sustaining a healthy work environment as a criterion in each nurse leader's performance appraisal. Nurse leaders must demonstrate sustained leadership in creating and sustaining a healthy work environment to achieve professional advancement.

- Nurse leaders and team members mutually and objectively evaluate the impact of leadership processes and decisions on the organization's progress toward creating and sustaining a healthy work environment.

NOTE

These standards were developed for use in the United States of America based on evidence from the American experience. Applicability of the standards for other countries and cultures has not been established. The American Association of Critical-Care Nurses requests that any experience and evidence derived from application of these standards in other countries and cultures be communicated in writing to the association.

REFERENCES

American Association of Critical-Care Nurses. (2005a). *AACN Standards for establishing and sustaining healthy work environments: A journey to excellence.* Aliso Viejo, CA: American Association of Critical-Care Nurses.

American Association of Critical-Care Nurses. (2005b). AACN Standards for establishing and sustaining healthy work environments. *American Journal of Critical Care, 14,* 187–197.

American Nurses Association. (2001). *Code of ethics for nurses with interpretive statements.* Washington, DC: American Nurses Publishing.

Back translation. (2007). Retrieved May 5, 2007, at http://www.asiamarketresearch.com/glossary/back-translation.htm

Greiner, A. C., and Knebel, E. (2003). *Health professions education: A bridge to quality.* Washington, DC: National Academies Press.

Hart, K. A., Ulrich, B., Lavandero, R., Woods, D., Leggett, J., and Taylor, D. (2007). Critical care nurses' work environment study: Implications for recruiters. *NAHCR Directions,* in press.

Institute of Medicine. (2001). *Crossing the quality chasm: A new health system for the 21st century.* Washington, DC: National Academies Press.

The Joint Commission. (2007a). Sentinel event. Retrieved April 27, 2007, at http://www.jointcommission.org/SentinelEvents/

The Joint Commission. (2007b). Sentinel event statistics. Retrieved April 27, 2007, at http://www.jointcommission.org/SentinelEvents/Statistics/

Kerfoot, K. M., and Lavandero, R. (2005). Healthy work environments: Enroute to excellence. *Critical Care Nurse, 25*(3), 72–71.

Maxfield, D., Grenny, J., McMillan, R., Patterson, K., and Switzler, A. (2005). Silence kills: The seven crucial conversations in healthcare. Provo, Utah: VitalSmarts.

McCauley, K., and Irwin, R. S. (2006a). Changing the work environment in intensive care units to achieve patient-focused care: The time has come. *American Journal of Critical Care, 15*, 541–548.

McCauley, K., and Irwin, R. S. (2006b). Changing the work environment in intensive care units to achieve patient-focused care. *Chest, 130*, 1571–1578.

McCauley, K. M., Barden, C., Lavandero, R., and Woods, D. (2007). The American Association of Critical-Care Nurses: Establishing and sustaining healthy work environments. In Mason, D. J., Leavitt, J. K., and Chaffee, M. *Policy and politics in nursing and health care.* 5th edition. Philadelphia: Elsevier.

Patterson, K., Grenny, J., McMillan, R., and Switzler, A. (2002). *Crucial conversations: Tools for talking when the stakes are high.* Hightstown, NJ; McGraw-Hill.

Patterson, K., Grenny, J., McMillan, R., and Switzler, A. (2004). *Crucial confrontations: Tools for resolving broken promises, violated expectations, and bad behavior.* Hightstown, NJ: McGraw-Hill.

Shirey, M. R. (2006). Authentic leaders creating healthy work environments for nursing practice. *American Journal of Critical Care, 15*, 256–267.

Thomas, D. (2003). *The ethics of choice: The handbook.* Omaha, NE: David Thomas.

Triola, N. (2006). Dialogue and discourse: Are we having the right discussions? *Critical Care Nurse, 26*(1), 60–66.

Ulrich, B. T., Lavandero, R., Hart, K.A., Woods, D., Leggett, J., and Taylor, D. (2006). Critical care nurses' work environments: A baseline status report. *Critical Care Nurse, 26*(5), 46–57.

Ulrich, B.T., Woods, D., Hart, K.A., Lavandero, R., Leggett, J., and Taylor, D. (2007). Critical care nurses' work environments value of excellence in Beacon units and Magnet organizations. *Critical Care Nurse, 27*(3), in press.

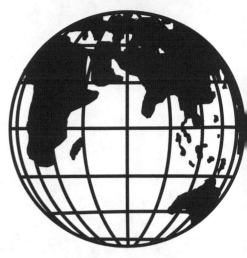

CHAPTER 6

MUTUAL RECOGNITION AGREEMENTS: SOME HEALTH POLICY AND PROFESSIONAL PRACTICE IMPLICATIONS

TOM KEIGHLEY, FRCN, RN, a Hons, DN, RCNT
GRAN CRUZ DE ASCOFAME, DIP HE THEOLOGY

While Mutual Recognition Agreements (MRAs) might not be the subject of discussion over coffee, their development is one of the major innovations of political life in recent decades. Because they happen at a supra-national level, are used by national politicians to explain away significant and often unpopular policies, and are monitored and implemented by remote and unseen bureaucrats, this is no surprise. While some of the larger frameworks for Mutual Recognition (MR) are increasingly well known, the recent agreements between the European Union (EU) and the United States (US) break new ground in a number of ways. In addressing this, I shall place the developments in the wider international context. The training and education of nurses will be used as the focus through which to examine the developments. The wider healthcare policy implications will also be addressed briefly.

EU-US AGREEMENTS

Discussions between the EU and the US were established as an annual event in 2000. The visit of President Bush to Vienna in 2006 saw the signing of a declaration to continue work on MR between the two national groupings. The declaration covers a number of trade and service areas. However, one section in particular is of significance for all professions.

> Improve the quality of transatlantic student mobility by promoting transparency, mutual recognition of qualifications and periods of study and training, and, where appropriate, portability of credits (Art. 3, section 3b—Council of Europe, 2006).

While the agreement refers to "renewing a programme of cooperation in higher education and vocational education and training," it goes significantly beyond this. Students could win sponsorship to study on opposite sides of the Atlantic in numerous ways. These are well known and much used. However, this is the first time that "mutual recognition of qualifications" has been referred to in such an explicit way. In the Annex, where the meat of all such agreements is to be found, under the heading of Action 3—Policy-oriented measures, is the following:

> The Parties may provide financial support to multilateral projects involving organizations active in the field of higher education and vocational training with a view to enhancing collaboration between the European Community and the United States as regards the development of higher education and vocational training. Policy-oriented measures may include studies, conferences, seminars, working groups, benchmarking exercises and address horizontal higher education and vocational training issues, including recognition of qualifications.

Of particular significance here is the reference to vocational training, as this covers all the healthcare professions, amongst others, and therefore by implication, the largest of them, nursing. Should this lead to an MRA, it will make it the largest in the world. The others currently in existence are as follows:

1. The EU

2. Trans-Tasman (excepting western Australia)

3. Caribbean Community and Common Market

4. Internal MRAs between the US and Canada

5. Eastern, Central, and Southern African College of Nursing

Work in progress includes the following:

1. North American Free Trade Agreement (NAFTA)

2. Mercocities Network (MERCUSOR)

3. Association of Southeast Asian Nations (ASEAN)

These developments are so important that global bodies like the International Council of Nurses (http://www.icn.ch/matters_mra.htm) and the regulatory forum of the Organisation for Economic Co-Operation and Development (OECD) are monitoring them. Increasingly, a sense exists that the future of nursing and other professions are being deeply influenced by patterns of training and practice that are not wholly home grown and that reflect the internationalization of healthcare delivery. The work between the EU and the US is ongoing with a further document having been produced in 2007 (Framework, 2007). This is of interest for its focus on regulation, a phenomenon of concern, because regulation is one of the controlling factors in the process of MR.

THE EUROPEAN EXPERIENCE

While it is a truism to say the world is getting smaller, Europe is expanding. Table 6.1 tells a story of marked expansion as well as indicates the desire of non-EU countries to be aligned with it. Full alignment means compliance with over 4,500 directives, legal acts that have to be passed into national law and then implemented to an agreed standard. Accession to the EU can be achieved only when these legislative acts have been transposed into national law and a timetable for implementation has been agreed to. A number of these directives, known historically as the Sectoral Directives, apply directly to healthcare professions. They are powerful tools for establishing a baseline of training for the professions while allowing the individual countries to go beyond if appropriate. While this can sound constraining, for countries emerging from the restraining culture of communist regimes and still striving to achieve western European standards in many fields of civic life, the directives have been an invaluable way of ensuring that local politicians and indeed other professions can be influenced to implement changes that can appear counter-cultural.

TABLE 6.1. COUNTRIES INVOLVED IN ACHIEVING DEGREES OF COMPLIANCE WITH EU REGULATIONS.

Members of the EU pre-2004	Countries that joined in 2004	Planned accession 2015
Austria	Cyprus	Turkey
Belgium	Estonia	*Other European countries*
Denmark	Hungary	*working to achieve areas of*
Finland	Latvia	*compliance*
France	Lithuania	Byelorussia
Germany	Malta	Moldova
Greece	Poland	Russia
Ireland	Slovenia	Ukraine
Italy	Czech Republic	*Non-European countries*
Luxembourg	Slovak Republic	*working to achieve areas of*
Portugal	*Countries that joined in 2007*	*compliance*
Spain	Bulgaria	Algeria
Sweden	Romania	Egypt
The Netherlands	*Countries working towards*	Israel
United Kingdom	*accession in 2011*	Jordan
European Trade Area	Albania	Lebanon
(who comply with EU	Bosnia-Herzegovina	Libya
directives)	Croatia	Morocco
Liechtenstein	Macedonia	Palestinian Authority
Norway	Serbia and Montenegro	Syria
Switzerland		Tunisia

NURSING DIRECTIVES

The nursing directives have a long history. Discussions in the EEC Council of Ministers in the 1960s led to the formulation of the directives, which became law in 1977. Further amendments have been agreed to, and a new directive has come into force that combines the existing ones (EU Parliament and Council, 2005).

Therefore, for nearly 40 years, the countries within the EU and those joining them have been working within these frameworks. They have provided structures that have ensured the development of the profession and protected both the quality of education and practice, while bringing into place systems to ensure the safety of patients. The following summarise the requirements:

- Ten years of basic education, attested by the acquisition of an appropriate diploma or certificate or an entry examination. (In reality this is moving towards being 12 years.)

- A course length of at least 4,600 hours and 3-years' duration.

- A division in training hours with theoretical instruction accounting for no less than one third of the course (1,533 hours) and clinical instruction representing no less than one half (2,300 hours).

- The subject of nursing to be taught by nurses, and clinical practice to be based in clinical settings, which must include primary care and where the supervision of the student is by another qualified nurse.

- The establishment of a regulatory function that:

  - Protects the title of "nurse."

  - Ensures the right of establishment of nurses, that is, they can work independently in a self-employed capacity.

  - Includes mechanisms for the registration of all qualified nurses and has the legal authority to discipline nurses and review the nature of their training.

To support this framework the Annex makes clear the basic content of nurse training. Broadly this includes:

- Knowledge of the sciences of nursing.

- Knowledge of the nature and ethics of nursing.

While this ensures sufficient breadth of coverage for nursing practice, the depth of coverage varies. Currently, entry onto the register is associated with an academic award. This varies between countries from diploma through degree and on to master's programs. This has occurred in parallel with the transition of nurse training from schools attached to hospitals over to universities and other centres of higher education. The transition has not occurred without debate.

BOLOGNA DECLARATION

From the late 1980s onwards, discussions emerged about the variation in the quality of the awards from different universities and in different subjects. Indeed, it was impossible to ensure that an Honours degree in one university department was comparable to the same award in another department of the same university. This resulted in the development of another system of mutual recognition.

Signed in 1999 to be implemented by 2010, the objective of the Bologna Declaration is to adopt across the EU, and many other signatory countries in Europe, a system of easily comparable degrees (European Higher Education, 1999). It is to be a system with two main cycles: under- and post-graduate. First cycle degrees will apply to the EU labour market as an appropriate level of qualification. The second cycle will lead to the masters and doctorate degree. Compliance with the declaration is open to EU and non-EU European countries. Critically, it legitimates academic training as an entry gate into professional practice, something that professions like nursing have long been seeking. Significantly, nurse education is now available at higher education level in all EU countries, even in France and Germany where resistance to the move has been greatest. Implementation of the Bologna Declaration plays into the knowledge debate by giving value to higher education, life-long learning, and research-based practice, all of which strengthen professions like nursing. Unsurprisingly, nursing is one of the professions specifically identified as part of this initiative.

The work is based on the creation of a system of transferable education credits, such as the European Credit Transfer System (ECTS). Through this, it is hoped that the mobility of the workforce will be improved further. It is also anticipated that European cooperation in education Quality Assurance (QA) will help to develop comparable criteria and methodologies and further, that curricular development, inter-institutional cooperation, mobility schemes, and integrated programs of study, training, and research will expand. It is in this context that the Berlin Conference of European Higher Education Ministers in 2003 (Realising the European Higher Education, 2003) raised questions about how to explore the U.S. quality experience.

The consequence of the declaration has been that centres of higher education have developed the ECTS to look like this:

1. One credit of education = 10 learning hours.

2. Modules are a minimum of 10 credits, but almost universally 20.

3. It is usual in full-time education to complete 120 credits per academic year.

Levels of education have also been determined. They are as follows:

- Level 1 = Certificate

- Level 2 = Diploma

- Level 3 = Degree

- Level 4 = Master's

This is all part of the EU free-movement agenda, the *acquis communautaire*. It rests on the development of a shared understanding of what competencies are and how to develop them and is underpinned by a common language or terminology that permits developments to be shared and implemented. The fact that nursing is at the centre of this is of real political and social significance.

IMPLICATIONS OF MRAS

The EU experience, focused on MRAs in nursing work, is of relevance for other countries. An MRA is a step toward globalizing the workforce. The impetus behind many of the existing agreements, and those being developed, is to make it easier for qualifications to be recognized and for the holders of the qualification to follow their profession in an ever greater number of international settings. It is also felt that the national (and in some settings, regional and local) constraints infringe an individual's rights to free movement. Conversely, the argument runs that nations will benefit from this sort of movement because it responds to the internationalization of markets. The inclusion of the free movement of healthcare services in the World Trade Organizations discussions underlines this.

Despite the close relations between the US and Europe, and the fact that a not insignificant number of European nurses spend some part of their nursing career in the States, nurses from the EU do not have automatic recognition in the US, and similarly, nurses from the US do not have automatic recognition in the EU. When comparing the education systems for nurses, it is clear why. The basis for training in both continents is radically different. Some may argue that the patterns of healthcare delivery are also different, but that is not stopping massive recruitment investment by U.S. concerns in the EU. A significant degree of movement is occurring internationally, as Mireille Kingma has recently recounted (Kingma, 2005). This is being determined by a difference in living standards, degrees of personal freedom, and economic opportunity. It has always happened to a certain extent. This time it is effecting healthcare and nursing in particular. This is why MRAs are becoming of real interest.

If there are strong personal drivers for this to happen, what are the political influences? In all the world's "developed" countries, health is on the agenda of politicians, put there by electorates that are concerned about access to services, the costs of care, and the quality of health services available to them and their loved ones, in particular ageing relatives. While the media carry stories about miracle cures and politicians know that there are votes in promising ever better healthcare, the key variable is the nursing workforce. Researchers like Ann Marie Rafferty and Linda Aiken have demonstrated for some years now that the single greatest factor effecting patient outcomes is the level and quality of education nurses have (McKee, Aiken, & Rafferty, 1998; Clarke & Aiken, 2003). The overriding problem is the shortage of nurses. The promises of politicians cannot be delivered because of the human resources issue. At this point the political and personal drivers become united. A wish to migrate meets a wish to import. Hence, the mass movement of nurses being witnessed today—Commonwealth nurses to the UK, Indian nurses to the Arab countries of the Middle East, Asian nurses to Australia, and nurses from all over the world to the US.

MRAs begin to address this. They rest on an agreement at a national or supra-national level, which means that the regulatory bodies in a country may legally recognize a qualification obtained from outside of its borders and so grant practice rights. To do this effectively, the regulatory body from which a nurse comes must at the very least have access to the training records, be able to vouch for the qualification held, and indicate that the person is in good standing in that country. Equally, the regulatory body in the country receiving the application must be in a position to receive and act on this data. This can be difficult when language and cultural issues intervene.

An MRA removes the need for the receiving country to do the hard work of individual assessment. In the presence of an MRA the regulatory body takes the assertion of its sister body at face value and acts upon it. Meanwhile, individuals have to undertake to follow the professional codes of the new country and not simply behave as if they were still under the regulation of their home country. This highlights the significance of how developments have evolved in the two latest agreements between the EU and the US. First, the idea of an MRA is sanctioned, and then the role of regulation is examined.

MRAs challenge notions of individual national sovereignty. Equally, they cloud some key fiscal issues. When individuals who have been trained at the expense of one country take their expertise abroad, the question of recompense does not arise. Should it? If nursing is the key variable in achieving successful healthcare outcomes, shouldn't a nation be paid back in some way for the lost investment? Equally, it is possible to ask why it is that politicians are not prepared to make sure that nurses are paid enough to ensure that they would stay in their homeland. While the answer may be that politicians will always go for the short-term option, deeper issues also emerge. If in the case of nursing the gender was male, would there be a different response to the challenge? Ever since the rape of the Sabine women, it has always been easier to accept the relocation of women across otherwise uncrossable borders.

A further issue to be addressed is patient safety. At one level, this has been addressed through language skills courses and bridging courses to fill competency deficits. However, behind it is a more significant development. With the vast majority of nurse publications being in English and both the percentage and volume increasing, English is becoming the de facto language of the nursing profession, as it is with other professions, so much so that schools of nursing all over the world now teach nursing in English alone. This benefits the English-speaking nations, but adds another burden on those nations least prepared for such challenges. The healthcare implications of facilitating the movement of nurses for the countries that they are leaving have yet to be fully identified. But its effect socially will not be insignificant on families left behind and institutions stripped of such talented and energetic individuals. It cannot be that the right to healthcare by nurses is limited to the richer countries.

CONCLUSIONS

It is difficult not to conclude that the nursing profession is moving into an era of MRAs. Not only do they redefine the way in which recruitment and the movement of the workforce occur, but also they challenge historic assumptions about what it means to be a nurse in any given country. The challenge in central Europe as those countries have joined the EU has been how to change a training system based on the gymnasium model where training for nursing and other professions started at the age of 14 years. A full-scale MRA between the EU and US would challenge fundamentally the system of community college training in the US as well as the balance of theory and practice in other, more eminent centres of education and training. The question to be faced is whether the benefits would outweigh the deficits.

One thing is certain, the degree of movement in the nursing workforce will remain high. In the light of that, it is essential that a much wider understanding of MRA be developed. It calls for significant reform of the functioning and capacity of the regulatory bodies in many countries and states. Unpopular as it might be, it also requires more investment in the regulatory function. Professional regulation is an area of significant specialism, but attractive to only a small number of people. The profession needs to be helped to wake up the challenges that lie ahead and begin to develop its thinking about the nature of training and the maintenance of its workforce. As John Donne wrote when Europe was the whole world:

> *No man is an Island, entire of itself; every man is a piece of the Continent, a part of the main; if a clod be washed away by the sea, Europe is the less, as well as if a promontory were, as well as if a manor of thy friends or of thine own were; any man's death diminishes me, because I am involved in Mankind; And therefore never send to know for whom the bell tolls; It tolls for thee.* (1624)

The italics are in the original, thus signaling what Donne thought was important. It is just as important for us, here, and now.

With thanks to Thijs van Ormondt, Law Online, Leiden, NL, for advising on the completion of this chapter.

REFERENCES

Clarke, S. & Aiken, L. (2003). Failure to rescue. *American Journal of Nursing.* Jan. 103(1): 42–47.

The Council of Europe. (2006). Council Decision on the signature of the Agreement between the European Community and the United States of America renewing a programme of cooperation in higher education and vocational education and training. Brussels, 23 May 2006, Institutional File 2006/0061 (CNS).

Donne, John. (1624). Meditation XVII from Devotions upon Emergent Occasions.

EU Parliament and Council. (2005). Recognition of Professional Qualifications, Directive 2005/36/EC. EU Parliament and Council: Brussels. 7th September.

The European Higher Education Area: Joint Declaration of the European Ministers of Education convened in Bologna on the 19th of June 1999. Universita degli Studi di Bologna, 1999.

Framework for Advancing Transatlantic Economic Integration between the European Union and the United States of America. 30 April 2007

McKee, M., Aiken, L., & Rafferty, A. (1998). Organisational change and quality of health care: an evolving international agenda. *Quality in Health Care*. Mar. 7(1): 37–41

Kingma, M. (2006). Nurses on the move—Migration and the global health care economy. Ithaca, NY, Cornell University Press.

Realising the European Higher Education Area—Contribution of the European Commission. Berlin, 18/19 September 2003.

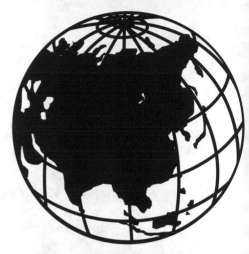

PART III

SUCCESS MARKERS

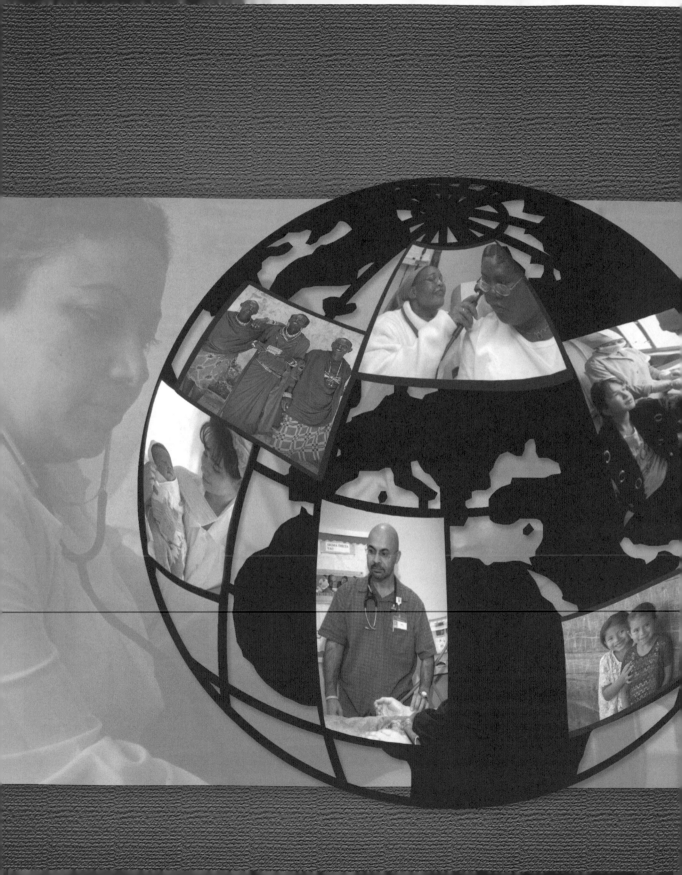

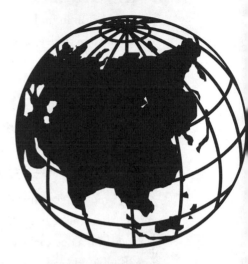

CHAPTER 7

LEADERSHIP ALLIANCES AND DIVERSE RELATIONSHIPS

SHEILA A. RYAN, PhD, RN, FAAN
MAJEDA MOHAMMED EL-BANNA, PhD, RN

Globalization presents challenges and opportunities for nurses and nursing. Lee (2000) defines globalization as a process that is changing the nature of human interaction across a wide range of spheres, including economic, political, social, technological, and environmental. Likewise, globalization is changing the face of healthcare delivery at home and abroad. International partnering facilitates cultural awareness, enhances educational programs, and results in personal and professional growth.

This is a story of a successful partnership developed between the University of Nebraska Medical Center College of Nursing (UNMC CON) and Alzaytoonah Private University School of Nursing (APU-SON) in Amman, Jordan. The partnership is a model program and may be replicated in other regions of the world. Principles of successful partnership are highlighted as they unfold in the story.

PRINCIPLE

The story began in mid 2003, when UNMC CON was about to graduate one of its most successful doctoral students, MJ, who planned to return to her native country of Jordan when she finished her studies. She was the recipient of the national Oncology Nursing Society's (ONS) best dissertation award for her nursing research with bone marrow transplant patients. She was not only a brilliant nurse researcher; she was compulsive about delivering excellence in everything she did. When she arrived in Omaha, she had never used a computer nor had she heard of American Psychological Association (APA) style. She quickly realized that she had to master both the computer and the style to be successful; she did this within a few months.

MJ's mother accompanied her to Omaha to assist with childcare for MJ's 2-year-old son and her about-to-be born daughter. MJ's husband, who supported her career throughout their marriage, was a doctoral student in international finance at the same time in a neighboring state, Kansas. He was sponsored by his bank employer from Amman to this specific university and expected to return upon completion within 4 years. MJ chose Nebraska for her research studies over a closer program due to the strength of the Omaha Medical Center's transplantation program with cancer patients. They saw this time as one of opportunity for them both, even though they were aware that strains and difficulties were inevitable.

RELATIONSHIP BUILDING

Identification of appropriate partners is essential to the success of a relationship. In international endeavors, we may locate our partners through exchange programs, sister city relationships, or hospital-based initiatives. In all cases, several principles of relationship building prevail. Some principles are detailed here; others applicable to process and challenges follow.

PRINCIPLE #1

Work with brilliant, highly motivated, and passionate professionals.

During MJ's studies, the UNMC CON Director of International Programs (DIP) was invited to submit a proposal to improve nursing education in Iraq. An existing relationship helped, thanks to a former medical resident at University of Nebraska Medical Center (UNMC). Currently a United States (US) Army director of health professions' education, the former resident communicated freely with his Omaha-based medical colleagues. Several phone conversations "from the war zone in the field" left the distinct impression that nursing and nursing education had fallen behind in the past 25 years under Saddam Hussein's regime. To illustrate the sense of urgency, about $20 million worth of intensive care unit (ICU) equipment was still boxed outside a tent because no one, neither doctors nor nurses, knew how to use it. The Army director's mission was to rebuild and staff three hospitals, and his invitation to us was to consider using our online teaching methods to partner with a nursing university in northern Iraq. He assured us that Iraq was "more computer-Internet wired than the entire state of Nebraska" and that online course delivery was highly feasible any place in Iraq. Furthermore, transportation into northern Iraq through Turkey and into the Kurdish towns was safer than in and out of Baghdad.

PROCESS

A decision was made to explore the possibility of creating a slight diversion in this opportunity by finding and using a safer nearby country such as Jordan to host the Iraqi nursing faculty and to train them on the online methods of the UNMC nursing courses. During my visit to Amman, I found Jordan to be a country of moderate politics and philosophy in a relatively advanced society. Visiting the major university's school of nursing revealed a primary interest in an American partnership "to provide them with well-prepared faculty, preferably doctorally prepared, to relieve their workload and high student clinical burden." While I visited several local institutions and foundations, it became apparent that even the Jordanians deemed Iraq too dangerous in which to travel or work. Once I returned to Omaha, I learned that my university benefits would not include travel deemed unsafe by the United States Department of State. A war zone is unsafe for travel. This made another principle obvious.

PRINCIPLE #2

Do not risk programs or faculty by expecting them to travel to, or participate in, unsafe conditions.

PRINCIPLE #3

Remember that learning is a two-way process, and local experts in-country should determine their needs.

When I returned from Amman, I immediately met with our soon-to-graduate nursing student, MJ, to inquire about the possibility of a partnering opportunity in Jordan. That's when I first heard MJ's passion—a passion bigger and deeper than for her research; it was a passion for her profession, her country, and for the possibility to advance nursing education throughout Jordan with our help. Seeking advice from the local expert—MJ—we identified a university that would benefit most from her dream and our assistance. She arranged an interview with the president of a new, private university in order to explore his interest in the proposed nursing program and a possible partnership with an American university's college of nursing. His answers were essential to our decision to move ahead with this shared partnership idea.

The president of the Jordanian University had a doctoral degree in nuclear physics from an American university; he wanted to have an American university partnership for each of his program schools. His dream included advanced preparation for faculty and new program offerings through the development and use of online learning technologies. He was open to joint faculty appointments, sharing learning technologies, regular travel, and finding the resources to improve the university's learning environments, and he held nursing in high esteem. The president's vision had all of the hallmarks of our shared strategies, a win-win in the making.

PRINCIPLE #4

Share mutual vision and goals but always start with what they say they need.

Much discussion focused on exploring our shared vision and goals. First, MJ and I agreed that we would develop a mutually shared vision and strategies. We would begin with an initiative that had a high probability for success, to ensure the successful launch of our partnership. Advancing nursing educational excellence through curriculum, research, and practice enhancements and advancing faculty preparation were priorities. As for the UNMC CON, the international program sought international experiences for students and faculty to learn from other cultures, while becoming world class in international outreach programs. A memorandum for shared strategies of the partnership would be articulated, identifying immediate, mid-range, and long-term goals and an implementation plan that clarified each partner's responsibility, measurable outcomes, and the financial exchange expected to achieve each goal outcome.

PRINCIPLE #5

Plan for here and now, soon—and build for later.

Perhaps, the most important aspect in our mutual planning was to start with the present—here—and respect our partners' identified needs. MJ was able to articulate immediately what she believed was the first strategy to be implemented: "We need a Learning Resource Center (LRC) just like you have here."

CHALLENGES

Common challenges related to international partnerships relate to funding, trust-building, and acquisition of supplies and equipment. We experienced these challenges in our relationship.

PRINCIPLE #6

Find a partner who can and will commit to finding its own necessary resources or will be willing to work together to solicit additional possible resources.

Previous experiences in Afghanistan taught us the lesson of caution to the "will and whim" of U.S. government aid to developing countries. Even with program grants solicited by government aid agencies, resources can be easily promised and broken in a single State of the Union address. Consequently, relying upon U.S. governmental aid was deemed too unreliable and saddled with a burdensome reporting process. Furthermore, experience taught me that preference was given to non-governmental organizations (NGOs) within the local beltway, owned by former employees who understood the right program-ese and requirements. On the other hand, it is fair to add that the government agency perception of universities is all too familiar, including high overhead, academic language, independent interventions, and prolonged time frames for implementation. Thus, finding financing for shared international partnerships requires funding opportunities unique to each partnership program. Relying on the basics of common expenses and revenue, such as tuition and travel budgets, constitutes a first-line strategy.

Another mechanism for gaining support for program investment is to conduct a "show and tell" tour. MJ was clear that a first strategy for nursing educational program enhancement was in the area of clinical instruction and, more specifically, to develop a skills learning environment much like she witnessed here in the US. She met with faculty at APUSON to discuss the partnership plans and concluded that a visit by her president and a board member with financial expertise would help them understand the investment necessary to replicate the LRC in Jordan. Together, we prepared a 3-to-4 page memorandum of agreement that was approved by all appropriate internal officials from both universities and that would be officially and formally signed by our two university principals during a joint meeting in Omaha. The signing ceremony would be followed by a tour of educational and clinical facilities, including the LRC. The officials would also experience our online course instruction for remote learners to pave the way for mid-range goals aimed at advancing faculty preparation and offering graduate level nursing specialty preparation.

Formalizing the relationship of partners is an important activity. The relationship is equal to, or perhaps more important than, the words in the contractual understanding. The document called for a 3-year time frame with an annual progress review and plans for renewal. International partnerships are only as successful as the relationships upon which they are based, and development of trust is tantamount to success. The formalization of the agreement engaged all levels of the UNMC enterprise, including legal and financial administrators. The UNMC Chancellor and Dean of the Nursing College met the president and board representatives from APUSON.

During this trip, we focused on sharing the clinical, educational and LRC tour resources. As MJ walked through the UNMC CON and LRC, she completed a needs assessment and inventory; the president and financial expert agreed to her requests. Our role involved assisting in the selection, acquisition, and maintenance of learning and simulation equipment to be ordered. Identifying the right vendor with the ability to provide delivery to Jordan and offer service with an acceptable maintenance contract was a time-consuming challenge.

PRINCIPLE #7

Understand the national and local infrastructure of needs, requirements, and approvals.

Private universities in Jordan are a new phenomenon. Resources for such entities are usually from philanthropic donors or owners. APU has five faculties (schools or colleges) offering baccalaureate degrees to approximately 5,000 students. Business and nursing are the largest programs, and both are growing in size and reputation. None of the programs offered a master's degree. In Jordan, the Ministry of Higher Education (MHE) approves all educational programs. In general, advanced faculty preparation is paramount to this approval. The MHE had not yet approved online education for credit, but the review process had begun.

The Jordanian nursing curriculum was organized similarly to the American undergraduate model and classes were taught in English. Master's programs in nursing were available in two public universities; a clinical specialty in adult medical-surgical nursing had recently been added. Undergraduate program requisites and prerequisites were almost identical; clinical hours were longer; clinical experiences were similar; but learning laboratory preparation for clinical instruction was non-existent.

A national Council of Nursing (CON) in Jordan had formed prior to our partnership; it had no formal jurisdiction. The CON's mission was to advance educational programs and curriculum of nursing to international levels and to evaluate and plan for accreditation and licensure mechanisms at international standards for the nursing profession in Jordan. One meeting occurred with the president of the Nursing Council before the partnership was formalized, and regular visits ensued.

SUSTAINABLE OUTCOMES

The partnership is approaching its three year anniversary and positive results are evident. First, APUSON has a large LRC composed of five fully-equipped simulation rooms to enable and enhance clinical instruction for students. MJ convened a three-day conference titled, "Clinical Instruction: Aspects for Success" for all APUSON faculty before the opening of the LRC. This conference was conducted in Amman, Jordan, by four instructors selected and invited from within the UNMC CON. Preference was given to those with expertise in the use of simulation in undergraduate nursing courses or clinical instruction.

A formal open house and ribbon-cutting ceremony was held in 2006 and included all university officials; the board of trustees; key leaders in nursing within Jordan's public, private, and military schools of nursing; and the Nursing Council president. Officials of all clinical agencies were also invited.

The highlight of the grand opening was the ribbon-cutting ceremony led by Princess Mona, the mother of King Abdullah of Jordan, who is also a board member and the patron of nursing and other caregivers in Jordan. Though she herself is not a nurse, her understanding, support, and encouragement for nursing is unsurpassed. The ceremony included individual briefings and explanations of simulation learning of critical-care and cardiac patients, obstetrical and delivering mothers, neonates and intensive-care newborns, and the elderly. Within weeks, the school was acclaimed to be one of the most advanced nursing programs in Jordan; the clinical simulation or LRC model was encouraged in all other schools of nursing.

One of the most significant outcomes was the faculty's growth and enthusiasm for clinical instruction following the 3-day conference. What the faculty first whispered, "Interesting but like playing with dolls," soon became a serious opportunity for them to improve the clinical learning for their students. The Jordanian faculty reported that this was one of the most important and valuable conferences they had attended and have requested that the same faculty return for clinical role modeling during which they would review and assess their clinical instruction styles. UNMC CON faculty also shared course outlines, syllabi, and tools for measuring clinical student performance at the request of Jordanian faculty. They wanted to improve their understanding of how clinical instructional objectives would integrate within the theoretical nursing course content.

It is apparent that a major success factor is the quality of the individual responsible for the partnership. When the nurse faculty leader has walked in two cultures and knows nursing and nursing education systems in both countries, she can more clearly see how one culture can improve the other. Then, the translation and language of needs, priorities, and plans for change are easier to understand, accept, and implement. Many American organizational work habits have been adopted at APUSON. Faculty now post office hours. Students are not permitted to smoke in the building. Students who need advisement for course changes must make appointments. Corridors are now quieter. Computers are on every faculty desk, and technical support technicians are available. Faculty departments are responsible for keeping minutes of meetings, and course changes and improvements are documented. The system of hierarchical decision-making is rapidly being replaced with decisions by a more empowered faculty.

Several faculty workshops or conferences were held in Alzaytoonah about nursing accreditation, its form and process. A "mock" self-study was prepared this year as a sample report to the MHE in Jordan with the assistance and advice of the American Association of Colleges of Nursing (AACN), which has expressed an interest in international accreditation. Accolades for the high quality of the nursing educational organization and its programs at APUSON were offered by the MHE. The AACN compared the APUSON program to many of the best programs in the US. MJ, the dean of the school of nursing, has been appointed to a newly formed national committee to develop educational accreditation processes for all disciplines in all universities.

Goals for advancing faculty preparation at the doctoral level are progressing. One APU-SON faculty member, enrolled in Omaha, Nebraska, at UNMC CON, is in his second year of study; another has been accepted for admission in the fall of 2007. Discussions about promoting bachelor of nursing (BSN) graduates directly into admission to the doctor of philosophy (PhD) program offers promise to increase the numbers beyond the current one or two applicants a year. All applicants require careful selection, advising, and assistance in the preparation for admission by the Jordanian Dean. Methods to assist Jordanian BSN graduates in preparing for admission into this program need to emerge, and additional financial resources will need to be identified.

The development of the clinical master's program in Jordan with clinical nursing specialty coursework through online learning opportunities has had limited success. The request to initiate a master's degree program in nursing at APUSON was initially denied because of a lack of qualified faculty at the doctoral (PhD) level. The MHE is continuing to study the possibility of approving online educational coursework but has not yet approved it. When approval has been granted, the plan is to enroll two or three Jordanian faculty in different online clinical nursing majors every year to expose them to the rigors of American master's level nursing curriculum and to increase their understanding of online learning methods.

The president of Alzaytoonah has demonstrated his interest in online learning technologies by purchasing the Blackboard software for course program management after consultation with our faculty. He has required each school in Alzaytoonah to begin faculty training in online course preparation and production. The dean of the nursing program has prioritized the creation of a Center for Arabic Nursing Education Excellence (CANEE) and plans to use online outreach methods to help other Arab countries advance their nursing programs if they choose to partner with Alzaytoonah. It is evidence of success when partnership is valued as a means to collaborate with, and reach out to, other new partners.

The dean at the APUSON in Jordan is critical to the success of this partnership. As the nurse leader of this partnership with Jordan, this new PhD graduate returned to Jordan with an American partnership plan in hand and soon was promoted from faculty and director of the partnership to department chair and then to dean of the nursing school. The original agreement protected one half-time of her time for partnership activities. Promotions limited MJ's time but enhanced her sphere of influence. MJ is the first Jordanian nurse to hold a PhD and to work in Jordan. Many doctoral level faculty are teaching in Jordan, but they are not Jordanian. They are migratory faculty from other Arab countries, primarily Egypt. They are great nursing teachers, but they receive higher pay including residence and travel support. They usually return to their homes during summer and holidays. Faculty contracts are only 3 or 4 years in length; foreign faculty prefer to return to their families in their own lands. Thus, development of a stable and committed faculty within Jordan is crucial to ongoing success.

OVERCOMING VULNERABILITY

Sometimes success breeds new vulnerabilities. MJ could easily be recruited away if adequate resources are not continued to allow for growth. For example, she can recruit Jordanian PhD faculty but must be allowed to offer competing salaries, including travel costs, and comparable workload. It may be necessary for the AACN to share its annual faculty salary comparison data across the US to help the Jordanian University president and board to understand the nature of keeping pace with readily available information on faculty salaries. In many countries, salary information is private; salary issues may reflect gender and culture. Yet, disclosure may support growth and enhance credibility within Jordan and throughout the Arab region. The partnership is in place and progress continues, but UNMC CON needs to be flexible to help find mechanisms for continued sustainability.

The partnership must find new avenues, such as publication and research, to help nursing faculty engage in scholarly activities. The MHE will judge these faculty qualifications before approving the Master of Science in nursing (MSN) programs. UNMC CON faculty research programs could be extended to gain comparative samples from our partner school, while concurrently teaching "hands-on" data collection by faculty and students. Preparation for these additional research activities will require additional conferencing and project team preparation by our research faculty. Travel costs need to be budgeted beyond the first agreement. Video streaming and phone conferencing are methods that could help facilitate these efforts. Time differences of 9 hours make planning more difficult but not impossible. Knowing that the weekend in Jordan is Friday and Saturday and the U.S. weekend is Saturday and Sunday also reduces access for shared work time.

We plan to explore partnering with national nursing societies such as the ONS and Sigma Theta Tau International Honor Society (STTI), who may welcome international research programs and meetings with our partner university to reach a larger national and international nursing audience. Timing is everything and while travel safety and security to this Arab nation present a challenge at present, the foreseeable future could be more favorable. The issue of travel security in an increasingly dangerous world reinforces the benefits of using information technologies. Online courses, phone and videoconferencing, web casting or archiving meeting sessions of American nursing scholarship or research presentations are now being planned and scheduled.

An international audience would relish the beauty, comfort, and engaging country of Jordan, surpassed only by the graciousness and warmth of the Jordanian people. The regional audience would embrace the opportunity to attend and participate in an international nursing conference.

THE FUTURE

What promise does the future hold? What is emerging? What work is yet to be done? Much of the future is in the hands of UNMC CON. Helping students and faculty in the CON grow with the partners in Jordan through exchanges, consultation, shared research, and online learning is a next priority. We need to better prepare our students and faculty for international learning experiences with a helping handbook. We are offering course electives in global health. We need to increase the opportunities for our students and faculty to engage in exchanges for professional nursing learning and sharing without losing time and credit for international travel experiences. We are expanding our understanding and knowledge of global health issues, and global health assessment strategies and measuring health outcomes are beginning to be formalized. We continue to identify appropriate faculty members who are able to work with international initiatives. Exploring the power of collaboration and partnering with other universities who are trying to develop global health educational elective offerings is underway. Discussions about a post-master's certificate program or a secondary major in global health are possible educational structures to be developed.

Global learning opportunities can enhance the institution with a planned "connection" strategy. Interdisciplinary goals, programs, and offerings maximize the potential reach for faculty and students alike. Mechanisms for integration of international "lessons learned" could take the form of shared seminars with all health professions programs or activities within the medical center and local community. A medical center web site with inventories of possibilities for faculty and students is currently being developed. Identifying local corporations actively engaged with international business partners and contracts could help leverage and share resources for expanding international opportunities with governmental aid in developing countries. The American Council on Education (ACE) published a series of works in October of 2006 aimed at improving institutional approaches entitled *Global Learning for All: The Third in a Series of Working Papers on Internationalizing Higher Education in the United States*. ACE outlines ways in which institutions may successfully advance internationalization. The series clarifies "internationalization at home" through programs and curricula; teaching-learning process; extracurricular activities; and integration with cultural and ethnic learning groups, initiatives, and activities. See Table 7.1.

"Internationalization Abroad" conceptualizes our thinking around moving people; moving programs; moving providers, such as campuses; and projects like capacity building, e-learning platforms, joint programs in education, and/or research programs.

International experiences are fundamental to learning cultural competence. Even though institutions of higher learning have taught, studied, and researched different ethnicities and cultures, health professionals still have knowledge deficits. As the National Center for Cultural Competence (NCCC) simply and clearly defines its goal:

> "As a culturally competent professional, I am capable of interacting with people who do *NOT* live like, look like, talk like, think like, believe like, act like…me."

REFERENCE

Lee, K. (2000). Globalization and health policy: A review of the literature and proposed research and policy agenda. In *Health development in the new global economy*. Washington, D.C.: Pan American Health Organization.

TABLE 7.1. UNMC INTERNATIONAL EDUCATION PROGRAM'S WEB SITE DATA COLLECTION FORM.

UNMC International Education Programs
Website Data Collection Form

Due by 1/22/2007
Return to John Adams
Chancellor's Office/Zip 6005

College, Institution or Unit: _____

Person submitting: _____

Program Name	Brief Description	Target Audience (Who participates?)	Schedule (When?)	Contact Person(s) Name Phone Email
Section A: International study and practice opportunities for UNMC students, faculty and staff				
Section B: UNMC study and practice opportunities for international students and faculty				

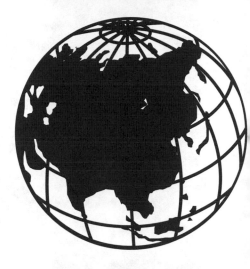

CHAPTER 8

ADVANCING EVIDENCE-BASED PRACTICE IN THE UNITED STATES AND ACROSS THE GLOBE

ELLEN FINEOUT-OVERHOLT, PhD, RN, FNAP

BERNADETTE MAZUREK MELNYK, PhD, RN, CPNP/NPP, FAAN, FNAP

Evidence-based practice (EBP) is using the best available evidence we have, whether that is clinical research or quality data, in combination with clinical expertise and patients' preferences and values to make decisions about care to produce the best outcomes (Melnyk and Fineout-Overholt, 2005). This process, occurring in the context of caring, allows for every clinical situation to be addressed in an individual manner so that these aspects of EBP are blended for the best outcomes for that patient or population (Figure 8.1). Considering that data-driven decision making has been our paradigm since day one, evidence-based practice was a natural fit for us. In addition, we believe in valuing and integrating clinical expertise and a clinicians' personhood, which leads to the best healthcare decisions. It is easy for us to be passionate about advancing EBP.

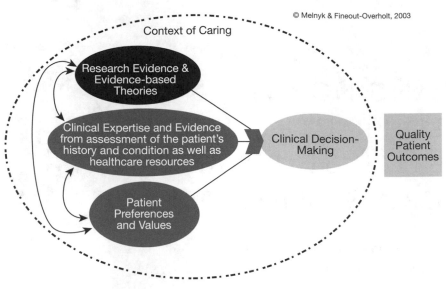

Figure 8.1. EBP conceptual framework.

Almost 20 years ago, we began this journey with a big dream to make a major positive impact on the healthcare and patient outcomes not knowing exactly where it would take us. We met in doctoral study and knew that, as a team, we could make a difference in outcomes, both at the point of care and in academia. We have pursued the dream of helping others to make a difference in their careers and with their patients, in large part through evidence-based practice. It has taken us to places that we truly could only have dreamed of when we started. Come along with us as we tell you our story.

"...for better or worse, our future will be determined in large part by our dreams and by the struggle to make them real."

—Mihaly Csikszentmihalyi

WHAT MAKES EBP A LIVED EXPERIENCE

The four sets of principles that we continually operate from are fairly simple. First, keep the dream alive and the vision fresh. Second, believe in the ability to accomplish the dream. Third, persist through the character-building times with sheer determination and persistence. Fourth, work consistently as a team. Adhering to these principles is what has enabled us to continue to work together to advance EBP and live our dream.

Keeping focused on the dream and believing in the ability to accomplish it are the first principles that we have found helpful in our efforts to advance EBP across the globe. In reading biographies of successful people who have made transformational changes, we learned that it is the dream that enables forward motion when "character-building" experiences arise. When part of the dream is squashed by circumstances or other factors, it is imperative to keep believing in the vision and the ability to accomplish it. The vision from the beginning was not "going global," but rather making a difference through advancing EBP and operating based on the adage "when opportunity knocks, open and walk through the door." An aspect of keeping the vision fresh is reframing what some might call obstacles, bad days, or barriers into more advantageous character-building opportunities. This framework enables us to discern how this opportunity will assist us in moving further toward the vision. Through the many character-building opportunities we have had in the past 20 years, it has sometimes been challenging to keep the vision fresh, but it also has been the definitive strong point in making our dreams become reality.

We also have found that persisting through the tough or character-building times is another key to achieving successful outcomes. So many individuals give up just before their dreams become reality. We persist until our dreams come to fruition. When we started an intensive effort to advance evidence-based practice in 1999, we were confronted by many well-meaning but skeptical individuals who told us that nursing would never embrace evidence-based practice and that it was no different than research utilization. We considered and weighed their admonitions with our belief in the dream. We kept focused on our vision, continued to believe, and persisted in our efforts, which enabled us to achieve the outcome.

The final key principle of working as a team may seem rather straightforward; however, we are two very different people. We come from different perspectives, different values in some cases, and have different approaches to getting work accomplished. We appreciate these differences and use them to maximize our strengths as a team. One of us has the primary role of being the big dreamer, and one of us has the primary role of process to make sure we achieve the dream. The differences that we experience could, at times, have created character-building opportunities for us—no one said that living the dream is easy. Members of a team are among other things: a) adaptable; b) collaborative; c) committed to the dream; d) communicative; e) competent; f) dependable; g) disciplined; and h) valuing of others' contributions, according to John Maxwell (2002). Members of a team trust one another. These characteristics are evident in how we approach our work together.

Teams are not always static, and we have had many wonderful people join and leave our team from time to time. That is the joy of a solid foundational core for the team; it allows for others to join and leave without the core being altered, thereby sustaining the efforts and advancing the work. No matter who we have had on our team at any given time, the uniting factor is that we all believe in the vision of advancing EBP to assist healthcare providers and patients in achieving the best outcomes. For example, when the president of Arizona State University, Michael Crow, embarked on a collaborative relationship with Dublin City University, we did not know we would have such wonderful collaborators as Joanne Cleary-Holdforth, Therese Leufer, Chris Stevenson, and Anne Scott with whom to advance EBP on the Emerald Isle. As team members, they have moved the efforts forward extensively, and we recently had the unique privilege of spending time with their faculty and nursing staff to teach EBP and to discuss how best to advance evidence-based care in Ireland.

"It is difficult to say what is impossible, for the dream of yesterday is the hope of today and the reality of tomorrow."

—Robert H. Goddard

THE PATHWAY TO MAKING A DIFFERENCE WITH EBP

Our joint EBP journey began in 1999. Dr. Bernadette (Bern) Mazurek-Melynk was appointed associate dean for research at the University of Rochester, part of a large academic medical center. With her experience as a nurse practitioner, she believed that the research-practice gap had to be bridged and that the key to success was evidence-based practice. Bern expanded the research center that she directed to include a main focus on evidence-based practice and needed an associate director as a close collaborator to help advance EBP throughout the academic medical center and community. She invited Ellen to join her as associate director to advance EBP in the acute care setting. Ellen had always based her practice on evidence and sought to help nurses evaluate outcomes, whether in academic, acute care or community health settings, so the fit was right. Thus, we embarked on this exciting journey, beginning with creating a vision for how we would accelerate what was then a very slow movement toward EBP in the nursing profession.

The first undertaking was a survey that was conducted within our medical center to assess the needs of advanced practice nurses regarding evidence-based practice. A strategic plan was then formed to begin mentoring staff in EBP. Part of the strategic plan also was to begin a national EBP conference, which was launched in 1999. The conference drew only 40 attendees. With that limited conference response, we were confronted by several well-meaning people who told us that nurses were not ready for EBP and that we should give up the idea and the work. However, we both believed in the vision and knew that we would eventually grow the conference to hundreds of like-minded attendees from across the US. We kept believing and persisting through the "character-building" times when most of our colleagues did not share our beliefs in the value of EBP.

Advancing Research and Clinical practice through close Collaboration (ARCC), our system-wide implementation model of advancing and sustaining EBP, also was conceptualized in 1999. We have spent the last 8 years gathering evidence from research to support the model and refining it to be useful in guiding the highest quality of sustainable evidence-based healthcare. The first step in the model is making a system-wide assessment to determine strengths and limitations of the organization in advancing EBP. Once determined, ARCC strategies are implemented to accelerate the pace at which EBP is implemented in the healthcare organization. A key ARCC strategy for system-wide implementation of EBP is that of an ARCC EBP mentor, most commonly an advanced practice nurse with in-depth knowledge and skills in EBP and organizational change. The ideal is to have EBP mentors at the system's level, the Advanced Practice Nurse (APN) level, and the staff nurse level to sustain best practice across the system. The ARCC EBP mentor works closely with direct care staff in implementing EBP, including outcomes-management projects, which our research has shown lead to stronger beliefs in nurses about the value of EBP and their ability to implement it (Melnyk, Fineout-Overholt et al., 2004). Subsequently, stronger EBP beliefs lead to greater EBP implementation. Another study that we have recently conducted indicates that the greater extent to which nurses implement EBP, the more group cohesion that they perceive. Through other research, it has been supported that higher group cohesion leads to greater nurse satisfaction, which should result in less nursing turnover rates at a time of a severe nursing shortage. Thus, one of our current dreams is that by 2020 all healthcare institutions across the globe will be employing advanced practice nurses as EBP mentors.

"They say dreams are the windows of the soul—take a peek and you can see the inner workings, the nuts and bolts."

—Henry Bromel

BUILDING THE CRITICAL MASS

One of the defining characteristics of an organization that is ready for system-wide implementation of EBP is a critical mass of clinicians with EBP knowledge and skills. Our energies have been intently focused in the past few years on building that critical mass across the globe. The joy of working with healthcare providers who desire to improve patient outcomes through EBP is that it is the same dream, no matter where you are living it.

The culture of each wonderful collaborator with whom we have had the privilege of working has enhanced the vision of assisting healthcare providers within the US and from across the globe to practice from the EBP paradigm. We have similarities that we all understand, and we have unique opportunities to reach clinicians in their culture to meet the needs of the peoples for whom they care. With the assistance of many, including Arizona Statue University (ASU) faculty such as Dr. Carol Baldwin, director of the Office of International Health, Scientific, and Educational Affairs at the College of Nursing and Healthcare Innovation; the Pan American Health Organization (PAHO); and Sigma Theta Tau International (STTI) we have enjoyed learning from all of our current U.S. and global partners, including Argentina, Chile, Colombia, Ecuador, Ireland, and Mexico. They have taught us that those who care about their patients can come together and make a difference in their own care and the care of those who they influence. We were privileged to work with Colombia and the Asociacion Colombiana de Facultades de Enfermeria (ACOFAEN) group, a faculty group that supports nursing educators, to advance EBP in South America. Everyone enjoyed this wonderful opportunity to work with educators and clinicians in Argentina who desired to establish EBP as a foundational aspect of nursing education. Some of our Hispanic colleagues from ASU, such as translator and epidemiologist Graciela Silva: our Argentinean hostesses Genoveva Avila and Maria Cristina Cometto; and our Colombian collaborator Maria Iraidis Soto S. helped us to live this dream and are continuing to live the dream with us. Scholars came from four different countries across Central and South America to join together to advance EBP and improve healthcare outcomes not only in their countries, but also across the Pan Americas.

> "Nothing in the world can take the place of Persistence. Talent will not; nothing is more common than unsuccessful men with talent. Genius will not; unrewarded genius is almost a proverb. Education will not; the world is full of educated derelicts. Persistence and determination alone are omnipotent. The slogan 'Press On' has solved and always will solve the problems of the human race."
>
> —Calvin Coolidge

HOW TO LIVE THE DREAM

The processes we used to live this dream have not always been consistent. We view this flexibility to engage different processes as strength. The consistent steps to the process have been very much the EBP process (see Table 8.1):

1. Determine what we really care about.

2. Find the evidence to answer it, through research, through data, through experience.

3. Keep the good stuff and use what doesn't work to teach us something.

4. Make what we've learned live in how we approach our work.

5. Assess and continually monitor our outcomes.

TABLE 8.1.   EVIDENCE-BASED PRACTICE PROCESS.

Step 0—Establish a spirit of inquiry

Step 1—Formulate the searchable, answerable question

Step 2—Find the best evidence to answer the question

Step 3—Critically appraise and synthesize the evidence

Step 4—Integrate the best evidence with clinicians' expertise and patient preferences and values

Step 5—Evaluate the outcome of implementation of evidence

It is not always easy to determine what it is we really care about the most. This step in the process cannot be engaged without considering the core values upon which one lives and practices. Family, faith, humor, and a good work ethic are values that underpin our efforts as we advance EBP. Often these values are in conflict with the demands that exist in global efforts (e.g., extensive travel to other countries). However, with these firmly established, what one is interested in can be more easily determined. We have found that these same core values allow us connections with our global partners that help in advancing the efforts because we all know that these values are givens.

Once we have determined the vision with our partners as well as what we all truly care about and exactly want to pursue as initiatives, we embark upon finding out what is necessary to inform these initiatives. Some of the informing factors we look for are research, cultural practices, inherent perspectives that exist in the healthcare systems within which the initiatives will live that will impact the outcome; and experience as to how things have worked in the past. All of these inform our decision making and action strategies to accomplish the outcomes.

In deciding what is good to keep or what perhaps has been viewed as character building and something to learn, we discuss each piece of "evidence" among our partners, and all perspectives are uniquely valued for their contributions. This is when we establish the outcomes we expect to find along the way and at the end of the initiatives. Dialogue, particularly on sensitive subjects, is a tool that we universally employ and have found to be invaluable in allaying any opportunity for misunderstanding that may stymie efforts to advance EBP.

Once we have had a thorough discussion, we work toward making the initiatives live, incorporating what we have learned from the "evidence." Sometimes, as with an EBP initiative, we have to change our plan in midstream, but that is the joy of having core values drive the work and having a solid set of principles that underpin the vision—change is viewed as an opportunity.

Finally, we keep tabs on whether or not we are getting the outcomes all of us have agreed upon from the EBP initiatives, whether that outcome is closer ties with our global partners, one facility that is closer to making EBP a cultural foundation, or one person who wants to become more of a leader in EBP.

THE PATH TO SUCCESS IS PAVED WITH OPPORTUNITIES FOR CHARACTER BUILDING

In framing our challenges as character-building opportunities, we have decided that we are truly characters. We enjoy the challenges, look forward to the problem solving, and love it when we achieve our vision and goals, despite the obstacles. We have learned that often one of the most persistent character-building opportunities comes from our own or others' expectations of "how things are supposed to turn out." When we are collaborating with our global partners, these expectations have offered us many opportunities to dialogue about how to best meet needs across cultures and countries while still maintaining the vision. Our global partners have the marks of those who move frontiers forward, the experience of having the wind in your face and arrows in your back. However, when they keep going and embrace the challenges, including language, culture, and time, as mechanisms to achieve the vision, good things happen.

Although some individuals have told us that they perceive the work that we do (e.g., making a difference, traveling to exotic countries, working with wonderful people) to be rather glamorous, we would like to dispel that myth. Often, the schedule kept and negativism encountered is very challenging. Sometimes the dream seems a little too big, until we remind ourselves to take the journey "one bite at a time." This motto has been a mainstay for how we have been able to make the dream live. We envision our work globally as a larger-than-life chocolate elephant, and right now, we are in the process of eating one small bite after another small bite, staying clearly focused on our dream.

"Should you shield the valleys from the windstorms, you would never see the beauty of their canyons."

—Elisabeth Kübler-Ross

HOW TO SUSTAIN DESIRED OUTCOMES OF THE DREAM

The outcomes of our dreams often are on a continuum. Some outcomes are very small, and some are so huge that it is, at times, fully challenging to comprehend them. When dreams get clouded or fears get bigger than the dreams, that is when progress will slow. At these times, we remind ourselves and help each other stay focused on our dreams.

What we would like for you to take away from this short journey with us is that you can do whatever your mind can conceive. The belief you have in your own abilities and those of others to achieve the outcome will influence how successful you will be in your efforts. So remember, stay focused on your dreams, believe in your ability to achieve them, persist through the character-building times, form an awesome team, and enjoy the journey. You can do it!

"When you want to believe in something, you also have to believe in everything that's necessary for believing in it."

—Ugo Betti

REFERENCES

Maxwell, J. (2002). *The 17 essential qualities of a team player*. Nashville: Thomas Nelson.

Melnyk, B. , Fineout-Overholt, E., Feinstein, N., Li, H., Small, L., Wilcox, L., & Kraus, R. (2004). Nurses' perceived knowledge, beliefs, skills, and needs regarding evidence-based practice: Implications for accelerating the paradigm shift. *Worldviews on Evidence-Based Nursing*. 1(3):185-93.

Melnyk, B. M. & Fineout-Overholt, E. (2005). *Evidence-based practice in nursing and health-care: A guide to best practice*. Philadelphia: Lippincott, Williams & Wilkins.

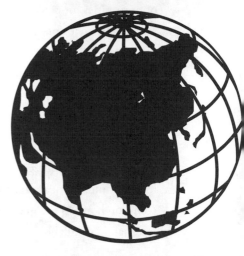

CHAPTER 9

CREATING COMMUNITIES OF INTERNATIONAL COLLABORATION

ANN MARIE T. BROOKS, RN, DNSc, MBA, FAAN, FACHE, FNAP

According to Rosen (2007), collaboration can be defined as "working together to create value while sharing virtual or physical space." Nurses are collaborators who recognize the importance and benefits in sharing knowledge, addressing common issues, and building capacity in nursing education, practice and research on a global scale.

Collaboration is an important process in creating global communities. Nursing has a long tradition of international collaboration through participation and leadership in international organizations, partnerships, consultation, teaching, and networking. Nurses have been risk takers, change agents, and activists in advancing nursing and healthcare's agenda, resulting in changes in health policy, new standards, and improved patient outcomes. Although the benefits of this work have been substantial, the international work of nurses has gone largely unnoticed by colleagues and international nursing and healthcare organizations. Some of this can be attributed to both a lack of visibility and a lack of evidence to demonstrate the impact of this work on health care outcomes. This situation may be about to change.

The recent increased emphasis on globalization provides nursing and other disciplines new opportunities for collaborative international work that can be assessed and measured. Success will require that nurses and other interdisciplinary groups share common visions, demonstrate coordination in problem solving, and maximize the use of human and fiscal resources in order to achieve optimal outcomes with expected sustainability of results. Access to and innovative use of technology will continue to provide invaluable support for communication and learning. The need for "ongoing connection" is critical to the success of working with others around the world. Nurses recognize the importance and benefits of working with others around the world.

This chapter focuses on five nurse leaders involved in global building activities working through international organizations. While their roles and accountabilities differ, they share a common bond in their commitment to excellence and to the advancement of nursing through international collaboration.

AMERICAN INTERNATIONAL HEALTH ALLIANCE

The American International Health Alliance (AIHA) was formed in 1992 to advance global health by helping communities and nations build sustainable institutional and human resource capacity. AIHA operates under various cooperative agreements and grants from the United States (US) and international donor agencies, including the United States Agency for International Development (USAID) and others. AIHA's approach offers partnerships and programs based on the philosophy that partners from abroad are more receptive to new ideas when they work with colleagues who face the same challenges in their day-to-day practice. Five key pillars serve as the framework for the work:

- Introducing new models of care and services
- Mobilizing communities for change
- Building sustainable capacity among healthcare practitioners
- Furthering the development of health-related professions
- Expanding knowledge through effective dissemination of successful programs

Nursing has been a vital part of AIHA's programs since 1992. Initial nursing efforts addressed improving the qualifications and status of nurses through individual partnerships, conferences, and focused programs. Hospitals and academic health centers from across the US applied or were recruited to participate in this partnership model approach. Interdisciplinary teams formed the core group of participants and essentially drove the agenda, goal setting, and coordination work. Partnership agreements were typically 3 years in length and provided resources for peer-to-peer visits, education, and the development of teaching materials. Frequently, organizations contributed additional funding or equipment as part of an effort to enrich the experiences or sustain changes in practice.

As a coordinator of a program in a large academic university health center, I experienced first-hand the rewards and challenges of working with nurses and physicians from Russia who were working with U.S. counterparts for the first time in their lives. The coordination and support from AIHA was invaluable and provided the needed coaching, facilitation, and cultural bridging critical to mutual goal setting and agreement on priorities. During our initial partnership efforts, we sponsored three different groups of nurses who stayed for a month at our organization expecting to return to their organizations with expert skill sets, improved ability to communicate in English, and an in-depth understanding of how to change their systems. While these goals were admirable and reflected a genuine commitment of nurses and the partnership team for improvement, it became critical to establish realistic priorities and strategies for baby steps that would lead to success in improvement in practice, education, and research in their organizations.

One of the most beneficial aspects of the partnership was the participation of American staff nurses in hosting and mentoring the groups of Russian nurses and physicians who came as part of the immersion experience. The common reaction following any visit by American participants was always, "I am so glad that I had a chance to learn more about what nurses do in Russia and what their educational system is like. I enjoyed teaching them about what we do, but I feel as if I gained much more than I gave because of what I learned about the barriers and obstacles they face every day. It is hard to imagine what nursing is like without talking to them about their patients, their leaders and peers, and their dreams for the future."

In recent years, because of reductions in AIHA funding and shifting health priorities, the number of funded partnerships in hospitals and other organizations in the former Soviet Union and Central Eastern Europe has declined. The current primary focus of AIHA is on building primary care networks and addressing the critical crisis of AIDS in Africa.

VIEWING AIHA THROUGH THE EYES OF:
SHARON WEINSTEIN, MS, RN, CRNI, FAAN,
PRESIDENT OF GLOBAL EDUCATION DEVELOPMENT INSTITUTE

Sharon Weinstein, a recognized leader and international expert, played a major role in developing AIHA partnership programs throughout the 1990s and the first part of the 21st century. As a subcontractor, she led AIHA's nursing initiatives and implemented the programs that created infrastructure and enhancements in education, practice, and processes.

DESCRIBE YOUR ROLE AND WORK WITH AIHA.

My work with AIHA began immediately after the dissolution of the former Soviet Union. AIHA evolved as a result of the efforts of major healthcare organizations such as the National Association of Public Hospitals (NAPH), the American Association of Medical Colleges (AAMC), the Voluntary Hospital Association (VHA), and Premier, Inc., an alliance of 1,800 hospitals and health systems. My role was to facilitate partnerships between U.S. hospitals and their counterparts in the new independent states of the former Soviet Union (NIS) and Central and Eastern Europe (CEE). Charged with responsibility for specific countries, including Ukraine, the Russian Federation, Uzbekistan, and Armenia, I worked with the U.S. and foreign partners to create work plans specific to their goals. Exchanges were planned to and from Eastern Europe, and healthcare leaders were chosen to participate in those exchanges. It was clear, however, that nurses were not always recognized as leaders. The existing infrastructure did not include a significant role for nurses and nursing.

I realized that our approach to fulfillment of partnership objectives should include a nursing initiative, and to meet this need, I created the NIS Nursing Task Force (NTF). The NTF membership included U.S. and foreign colleagues. As counterparts, they met at designated intervals to share practice, process, and education. The CEE countries emulated the NIS model, creating the infrastructure needed to ensure sustained growth.

HOW SUCCESSFUL WERE THE PARTNERSHIPS IN ADVANCING NURSING IN THE FORMER SOVIET UNION?

Nursing in the NIS has become a recognized profession. Defined roles and responsibilities, standards of practice, licensure, and more have created a respected profession, moving the nurse from middle level personnel to a position of status. Chief nurses of the Ministry of Health (MoH) were appointed and nurses began to lead the way in healthcare delivery and outcomes. As I look back at our accomplishments, I take great pride in the nurses we have mentored and taught. Graduates of the International Nursing Leadership Institute (INLI), members of Sigma Theta Tau International Nursing Honor Society (STTI), authors, scholars, and leaders—nursing is now a source of pride and a valued profession.

WHAT WERE THE FACTORS THAT WERE CRITICAL TO THE SUCCESS OF THE PARTNERSHIP?

Factors critical to the success of the partnership model included creation of relationships with those in power, committed U.S. partners, enthusiastic and dedicated NIS/CEE partnerships, and in-kind contributions.

HOW DID THE LEADERSHIP PROGRAM(S) ENHANCE THE ACHIEVEMENT OF GOALS?

The leadership programs facilitated the achievement of goals by providing skill sets essential to surviving and thriving in a changing environment. Learning Resource Centers (LRCs), information technology, and communication were key to successes. Armed with the tools needed to lead the field, nurses gained confidence in themselves and in their abilities. Negotiating for success, succession planning, and communications skills—these and more helped to create a new generation of nursing leaders for the future and beyond.

WHAT HAVE BEEN THE MOST SATISFYING OUTCOMES OF YOUR WORK WITH AIHA AND OTHER PROGRAMS?

The most satisfying outcomes of my work with AIHA and the NIS/CEE leaders have been the creation of a cadre of educators, practitioners, and leaders. To see a nurse with an 18-month education develop English language skills and continue her education to the doctoral level is so rewarding. To share the podium before the U.S. Department of Health and Human Services with one's counterpart from an NIS country is a profound experience. And to develop a fellowship program for qualified applicants further advances the profession. Graduates of the INLI program and fellows of our advanced program communicate with their U.S. colleagues on a regular basis. Strong friendships have developed, and alliances have been built for now and the future.

HOW WOULD NURSES WHO PARTICIPATED DESCRIBE THE LEGACY OF THE PARTNERSHIPS?

NIS, U.S., and CEE nurses who participated in these partnerships describe them as career development opportunities. Through these relationships, they have grown personally and professionally. Members of the original NTF continue to collaborate in many ways, creating new opportunities to involve their NIS/CEE partners. This truly is a legacy!

VIEWING THE WORK OF AIHA THROUGH THE EYES OF:

SHEILA RYAN, PhD, RN, FAAN, BOARD MEMBER, AMERICAN INTERNATIONAL HEALTH ALLIANCE

HOW DID YOU GET INVOLVED WITH AIHA?

I first got involved with AIHA through the Premier/Strong Memorial Hospital Partnership Program. Sharon Weinstein was the program coordinator for Premier and AIHA. Ann Marie Brooks was on the on-site coordinator at the University of Rochester Medical Center. As Dean of the School of Nursing and Chief of Medical Center Nursing, I sponsored many of the activities for the month-long nurse exchange program and supported faculty's participation in a wide variety of activities. At the start of the 2nd year of the 3-year partnership, I was honored to be invited to be the keynote speaker at the 25th anniversary celebration of a Russian School of Nursing. During this visit to Moscow and St. Petersburg, I had the opportunity to meet several deans of schools of nursing who were all physicians. I learned first-hand about the challenges facing nurses in the former Soviet Union. Shortly after that visit, I was invited to serve as a board member of the AIHA board and have served in that role for the past 12 years.

DESCRIBE HOW AIHA HAS CONTRIBUTED TO THE ADVANCEMENT OF NURSING AROUND THE WORLD?

AIHA was a leader in recognizing the importance of nursing to healthcare. They devoted considerable resources (both human and fiscal) to leadership development and improvement in clinical care. Partnership teams were interdisciplinary and the majority of projects were focused on improvement of patient care outcomes. Major conferences were organized and offered with simultaneous translation and materials provided that could be used by participants at their own organization.

Examples are numerous and reflect the passion and excitement of both U.S. nurses and partners. As a board member, I had the privilege of attending a number of programs as a participant and observer. The Leadership Institute (a year-long program) three times is an example of a project that far exceeded expectations and whose participants continue to thrive.

WHAT HAVE BEEN THE MOST SATISFYING ASPECTS OF SERVING ON THE BOARD?

It has been inspiring to be at the "birthing" of professionalism, to witness the depth of their hunger, curiosity, and effort for updating and enriching nursing education, practice, and research. Being the primary spokesperson for nursing has afforded me the opportunity to expand nursing's visibility within the AIHA programs. I serve as a consultant and resource to the AIHA leadership staff and have networked with nurses in other organizations about the work of AIHA.

WHAT ARE FUTURE ISSUES THAT NURSES SHOULD BE CONCERNED ABOUT BOTH IN THE US AND OTHER COUNTRIES?

Many issues of concern exist, but I think three that are most pressing are:

1. Workforce migration and immigration status

2. The needs of women and children

3. Emerging infections

While no easy answers to any of these issues exist, it is important for nurses to be at the table for dialogue and advocacy.

WORLD HEALTH ORGANIZATION COLLABORATING CENTERS

World Health Organization Collaborating Centers (WHOCC) for International Nursing have played an important role in the advancement of nursing practice, education, and research around the world. Thirty-seven worldwide WHOCCs in nursing and midwifery development are organized into a global network, with 12 located in the United States. The centers are based within schools and colleges of nursing. The centers receive this special designation through an application and rigorous review process that is administered and monitored through the Pan American Health Organization (PAHO), as part of the larger World Health Organization (WHO).

Representative leaders from three U.S. centers were interviewed. As experienced educators and nursing leaders, they provide valuable insights about the challenges facing nurse faculty and others in establishing and maintaining partnerships. Their reflections on both the professional and personal satisfactions gained from their work provide insights not usually accessible to nurses interested in international work. The range of projects and leadership roles provide evidence of how these and other nursing and midwifery development centers have improved the health outcomes, enriched the education and continuous learning of nurses, and fostered cultural competence and awareness for partner groups and beyond.

COLUMBIA UNIVERSITY
SARAH SHEETS COOK, DRNP, RN-CS, VICE DEAN AND DOROTHY M. ROGERS PROFESSOR OF CLINICAL NURSING, COLUMBIA UNIVERSITY SCHOOL OF NURSING

HOW DID YOU GET INVOLVED IN INTERNATIONAL NURSING WORK?

The faculty at Columbia University School of Nursing have always been interested in international work and committed to helping nurses improve the health of others. We became actively involved in the 1980s because of the interest that Dean Mary O. Mundinger, DrPH, had in international work. In addition, schools of nursing and hospitals from around the world continually contacted us to learn about what we were doing at Columbia in preparing nurses for advanced practice. They sent faculty from their schools to Columbia to learn about how to their nursing education programs and nursing practice in their countries. They were also interested in learning how to influence and advocate for changes in health policy in their countries. Initially, we worked with them on raising the level of basic nursing education and improving health practices in various countries. It was clear to us that our partnerships were producing substantial results in educating nurses and raising the status of nurses with their healthcare systems.

DESCRIBE YOUR INITIAL WORK.

Our initial work was in Sweden, Korea, the United Kingdom (UK), New Zealand, Denmark, France, and Armenia, and we individualized the programs to fit the learning needs, culture and resources available. For example, in Armenia we partnered with Americare and developed a program for pediatric practitioners and clinicians. We created teaching modules focusing on upper respiratory infections and diarrhea. These modules were then implemented throughout their healthcare system, resulting in positive changes in the care of pediatric patients. Through our international work, we learned about the WHO Collaborating Center designation and began the application process in the early 1990s. We received our initial designation in 1996, our first re-designation in 2002, and again in 2007.

WHAT HAS CHANGED IN THE WORK OF THE CENTER OVER THE YEARS?

We have become more opportunistic, focused, and selective about projects. I serve as co-director of the center and share this leadership role with Dr. Richard Garfield, who spends the majority of his time out in the field working with our partnerships. Our center's advisory board reviews all the proposals submitted and determines the feasibility of each project. Funding is always a concern, and we seek and receive monies for projects from both governments and private philanthropy sources. For example, we helped develop a program for training indigenous workers in Ceara, an underdeveloped state in Brazil, to augment healthcare delivery systems in partnership with the government and other agencies. This project that prepared non-professional workers was successful in improving child health status, vaccination, prenatal care, and cancer screening in women through the provision of services at the local level.

WHAT EFFECT HAS THIS WORK HAD ON YOUR CAREER AND YOUR ROLE AS A LEADER?

Our WHOCC is really a collaborative project and not about me personally, although I have been able to turn my personal interest into professional pursuits. A natural evolution has occurred, and most of us have been able to integrate our international work and nursing into our teaching and scholarship activities.

WHAT DO SEE AS THE GREATEST NEEDS IN INTERNATIONAL NURSING WORK?

Several needs exist:

a. Migration of nurses—It is ethically outrageous to drain countries of their nurses, and we need to address this serious issue on a global level.

b. Develop nursing leaders—Some level of basic nursing education and some type of advanced nursing education programs are usually in place in most countries, even ones considered "developing." However, they are not usually equivalent to basic and advanced nursing in the US, but programs are there. The trick is to find the programs and nuture/develop leaders so nursing can become an active and productive partner in improving health care globally.

c. Prepare faculty for practice; foster faculty to practice—Many nursing schools are staffed by faculty who are not current in practice. If more faculty members were aware of healthcare needs internationally, they might be better prepared to teach nurses who could undertake strengthening the nursing profession across the world.

How has your work influenced the education of nursing students at Columbia?

We expose our students to what we do internationally, and we are able to plant the seeds and provide opportunities for them to do international work. Students have been involved with our projects in Cuba, Dominican Republic, Sweden, Armenia, and Korea—usually graduate students, both at the master's and doctoral levels.

Lessons Learned

Projects always take longer than expected, even if all parties are in agreement!

We couldn't survive without e-mail! I have enjoyed my work, have learned a lot from my global colleagues, and am proud of our center's work and our shared commitment to others.

University of Alabama—WHO Collaborating Center on International Nursing

Lynda Harrison, RN, PhD, Professor and Deputy Director,
WHO Collaborating Center on International Nursing,
University of Alabama

How did the center get started?

The University of Alabama School of Nursing began its international work during Dr. Rachel's Booth tenure as dean. Dr. Booth and other University of Alabama administrative leaders established a partnership with Chaing Mai University in Bangkok, Thailand. For the first few years, the major activities were providing assistance in improving nursing and medical education standards and supporting nursing and medical research. In nursing, these activities led to the application for designation as a WHO Collaborating Center for International Nursing and expansion of activities to other parts of the world. Since the initial designation in 1993 and subsequent designations in 1997, 2002, and 2007, the goals and objectives (known as the general terms of reference) have become more specific, and outcomes are evaluated in relation to strategic goals identified by WHO for nursing and midwifery outcomes.

HOW DID YOU GET INVOLVED WITH THE CENTER?

I had been doing some international work, but I became really interested after I represented our center at the 2002 meeting of the global network held in Chicago. Dr. Naeema Al-Glasser chaired the meeting and motivated the group to move from the talking phase to the doing phase. She divided the group into tables of common interest. Each table was asked to brainstorm ideas about how they could take the WHO Collaborating Center strategic goals and work together to produce realistic and usable outcomes. Following that meeting, I became an active member of the workgroup trying to develop an online graduate research course. That meeting also led to my application for a Fulbright Fellowship to study in Chile. During my 6-month study period, I conducted a needs assessment for research of nurses in Chile and worked with others from the global network workgroup and nursing faculty in Chile to develop an online research course for our other partners.

HOW HAS THE WORK OF THE CENTER AND THE FACULTY IMPROVED THE HEALTH OF PEOPLE IN OTHER COUNTRIES?

A number of examples demonstrate how the center has made contributions toward improvement. The center provided the infrastructure to organize our international work and outreach. In the early years of the center, the faculty was primarily involved in working with partners on improving nursing education and faculty development. Improvement of health outcomes has been the result of better educated nurses and faculty.

As the center has expanded its activities, we have become more specific in our goal setting. This approach has resulted in identifying measurable outcomes and has enhanced our ability to identify priorities and set mutual goals with our partners. For example, our recent work in Latin

America has focused on the development of a manual on the international management of children. The manual provides specific approaches in determining the various levels of needs using standard assessment tools. This manual will be a useful and much anticipated tool for nurses and other healthcare professionals in the entire assessment, treatment, and evaluation process.

WHAT ARE SOME OF YOUR GOALS FOR YOUR RECENT RE-DESIGNATION?

Our new terms of reference include appointing an advisory board for the center, naming faculty as center clinical scientists, and continuing to focus on projects that improve the quality of life and patient care outcomes of various populations.

CAN YOU DESCRIBE SOME OF YOUR NEW PROJECTS?

The first is a collaborative project with nursing faculty from the University of Honduras School of Nursing and focuses on a Family Life Education Program. A PAHO faculty member visited Birmingham in the spring of 2007 and trained 25 Latino health care providers prepared to teach a 7-week course on drug prevention to parents of 10–14 year olds. In the summer of 2007, the same course will be offered to parents in Honduras. This partnership project with the School of Nursing in Honduras will assist in building strong relationships and serve as a model for further projects.

We are now planning for an International Leadership Program that will start in January 2008. This one-year program is an expansion of a 2006 Chilean Leadership Project from 2006. This program will start with a 3-week immersion course that will take place in Birmingham. The participants will attend English courses every morning and spend the afternoon in classes on leadership and project development. Each participant will bring a specific idea for a project and will work with a mentor assigned during the program to develop a project plan that will be implemented during the program period. The addition of the project will strengthen the commitment of the participants and their home organization to the journey of leadership development.

WHAT HAVE YOU BEEN IMPRESSED WITH IN YOUR WORK WITH YOUR PARTNERS?

I have been impressed with their resilience and commitment to excellence. Many of our partners carry significant workloads and experience technology challenges that we in the US are not accustomed to in our workplace. Access to resources is limited, and the economic disparity is substantial. I have found that our partners stay motivated and committed to achieving project goals despite challenges because they value the opportunity to advance nursing and improve the health outcomes of their people. The international work of the center has been a privilege, and all of us report great admiration for the "depth of human spirit and enthusiasm for excellence" that is alive and well in our partners and colleagues around the world.

GEORGE MASON UNIVERSITY
DR. RITA CARTY, PHD, RN, FAAN, PROFESSOR AND DEAN EMERITA, GEORGE MASON UNIVERSITY, PAST DIRECTOR OF THE WHOCC, GEORGE MASON UNIVERSITY, COLLEGE OF NURSING

HOW DID YOU BECOME INVOLVED IN INTERNATIONAL WORK?

I became interested in international work for several reasons. Because I lived in the Washington Metropolitan area, I was constantly exposed to the changing face of the landscape and enjoyed the diversity of the population. In addition, as a faculty member at George Mason University, I received frequent requests to host international visitors. I wanted to improve our ability to both understand and meet their learning needs.

Dr. Jessie Scott, an esteemed colleague, encouraged me and helped me by identifying strategies to increase my knowledge and my networking. Dr. Amelia McGloches, WHO Chief Nurse Scientist, also mentored me and provided opportunities for me to develop expertise in international work. As I expanded my knowledge and after I became Dean, I learned about the opportunity for establishing a WHO Collaborating Center at George Mason. We achieved designation in 1990.

HOW DID YOU GET THE FACULTY INVOLVED?

As dean and director of the Collaborating Center, I wanted as many faculty involved in the activities of the center as possible and created a number of opportunities. I also made it a priority to ask different faculty to participate in each new project so there would be broad participation and capacity building across the faculty group. Recognition was an important part of the process and seemed to be appreciated by faculty, students, and staff.

Discuss your election as secretary-general of the Global Network of WHO Collaborating Centers for Nursing and Midwifery Development in 2000.

Serving as the secretary-general and bringing the Global Network Center to George Mason University was an honor and a great opportunity to help others involved in international work. The center had been located at several other sites: the University of Illinois for 8 years, Korea for 4 years, and in Manchester, England. In 2000, when the directors from the Global Network voted for the center to move to George Mason, I became the secretary-general. I enjoyed serving and am proud of the achievements that we were able to accomplish. While the center was at George Mason, we were able to make significant progress in integrating technology into the center's work. First, we were able to create an online procedure for the election of the secretary-general, which allows for a smooth and efficient process selection and transition process. Second, we were able to build a web site with web links to other centers and other organizations within the WHO. Third, we were to secure approval from the director-general of the WHO for appointment of a nurse representative from the Global Network to the Global Advisory Group that reports to the director-general of the WHO.

What advice do you give other centers and those considered applying for designation?

I advise centers to establish an advisory community board, create titles for faculty and participants within the center to provide credibility and recognition for their work, and to be creative in seeking sources of funding.

Words of Wisdom

1. First do no harm! Do things for the right reasons and give partners and others who we work with the respect and attention that they deserve. Respect their cultures and their environments and work toward common goals.

2. Listen, listen, listen! Give those you work with enough time to hear what they are saying. Nurses from outside our country do not always have the experience that we have and may require more time because of language and the lack of experience in working with those outside their culture. If we don't take time to listen, we will be missing the opportunity to understand and build the trust needed to move forward and achieve mutually beneficial goals.

The five individuals presented in this chapter represent a wealth of knowledge and expertise in international nursing. They have created communities of collaboration through building trust, communicating respect, valuing and celebrating similarities and differences, and sharing knowledge to advance nursing education, practice, and research. Their courage, risk taking, and commitment to excellence have helped pave the way for all of us to continue building global communities of collaboration.

REFERENCES

Rosen, E. (2007). *The culture of collaboration*. SF: Red Ape Publishing.

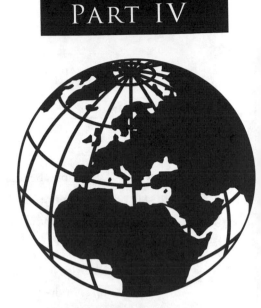

PART IV

COLLABORATION
SUCCESS STORIES

Perhaps one of the most gratifying developments from global partnering relationships is the accelerated advancement of the nursing
profession. While many of the initiatives described in *Nursing Without
Borders* recognized the importance of relationships from the outset of
collaboration, many of the partners did not realize how quickly results
would materialize and lives would be changed. The lynchpin behind the
success stories that follow has been the cooperative nature of nurses and
their strength and skills as nurse leaders. Collaboration denotes a two-
way learning experience. These stories tell it all.

1

The All-Ukrainian Nursing Association Workshop

Marjorie Beyers, EdD, RN, FAAN

Success can sometimes be measured quantitatively, but often, the most potent outcomes of an experience are not readily measured. This story is about an experience in the Ukraine, with nurses from every sector of the country who came together to learn about associations. The most potent outcomes were in four of the lessons learned, summarized as follows:

1. **Curiosity is a great equalizer.** It keeps the "foreigner" focused on learning how nurses in the Ukraine function, what their issues are, and how they conduct their nursing care services. Curiosity helps the in-country nurses focus on learning about nursing in another country, paving the way for shared experiences and continued learning.

2. **Nursing is universal.** There is something very special about nurses gathering to share their experiences. Nurses from different countries or sections of the same country all have common values and philosophy about the meaning of nursing for themselves and for their colleagues. The purpose of nursing unifies nurses in their commitment to the profession.

3. **The will to make things happen is an essential ingredient in any experience designed to achieve outcomes.** Another way to explain the will to act is the concept of intentionality (Lawler & Yoon, 1993, 1996). When people act intentionally, they develop the basic understanding of what needs to be done and how to proceed. They are open to learning what is needed to plan and act, intentionally, to achieve results.

4. **Nurses throughout the world practice in very diverse environments, but all provide a public service, subject to laws, regulations, and rules to protect the public.** The authorized functions of nurses, the resources they have to accomplish patient care, and the behaviors of nurses in practice are all affected by these laws, regulations, and rules.

These lessons learned comprise a retrospective view of what happened in Ukraine at the All-Ukrainian Nursing Association Workshop. My role was to present the United States (US) model for nursing associations and to work with the group in dialogue about applications to Ukrainian nursing. Held in Kiev, Ukraine, in August 2000, this workshop was sponsored by the American International Health Alliance (AIHA), with funding from the U.S. Agency for International Development (USAID) and participation from the U.S. Embassy in Ukraine. The workshop design was one activity in a broader initiative to assist in the continued development of nursing and patient care in Ukraine. Workshop participants included nurse leaders from hospitals in Ukraine, representatives of official organizations, and individuals whose positions involved work with healthcare organizations.

WORKSHOP DESIGN

Principles of adult learning were evident in the workshop design. Content was developed for 3 days of intensive learning, which began with formal introductions by officials from the AIHA Regional Director, Kiev; from the USAID; from the U.S. Embassy; and from Sharon Weinstein, the workshop principal and founder of the AIHA nursing initiative for the new independent states of the former Soviet Union (NIS) and Central and Eastern European countries (CEE).

The 3-day program was planned to begin with the Ukrainian experience, followed by a presentation on international organizations and then a presentation on the U.S. model of nursing associations with applications for Ukrainian nursing. This content provided the foundation for the remainder of the workshop. Brainstorming sessions were planned to allow participants time to think about the formal presentation content, to discuss their own experiences and the meaning of the content for them, and to discuss how a country-wide organization would serve nurses in the Ukraine.

Interactive learning methods were used for the remainder of the workshop. These learning methods included the first brainstorming sessions with reports of each group's findings, games to engage participants in teamwork experiences, and exercises to provide an opportunity to try out new ideas about their associations, all with the assistance of facilitators. Short, focused presentations on the resources available to local nurses, including the Nursing Learning Resource Center (NLRC), were interspersed with these interactive learning experiences. A site visit to the

Psychiatric Nursing Association headquarters provided an opportunity for nurses to visit a successful Ukrainian nursing association, to refresh, and to learn about the association's purpose, mission, and activities. Bringing together this nursing association with other specialty nursing associations throughout Ukraine was viewed as an asset to the continued development of nursing services in the country.

The final day of the workshop continued the theme of assessing needs and developing resources to meet these needs. The third workshop session centered on grant writing as a way to obtain resources for continued development. Content on action planning provided a vehicle for developing ideas and translating them to action plans, which then could be developed into requests for funding and support. Breakout sessions were planned to allow participants time to develop ideas and strategies for their future. Discussing next steps in the form of action plans involved not only conceptualizing the future, but also thinking about priority needs for development, resources essential to achieve action plans, and individuals and groups perceived to be key stakeholders and identifying activities to follow-up on the workshop experience. The final session for this workshop included a summary of the breakout session content and organization of this content into next steps for participants to take locally and country-wide.

Socialization was also planned for this group. Meal times were arranged to facilitate discussion and exchange among participants. Dinners were special events with opportunities for networking receptions, for sharing, and for appreciating each other. These dinners provided a time to "dress up," to enjoy food and conversation. The setting, a conference center in Kiev, provided the ambience for brief walks, for quiet time, or for small group discussions. Convening at the conference center was viewed as a special event by many participants, which was convenient, comfortable, and "their space" for the 3-day workshop.

WORKSHOP CONTENT

Workshop participants were generally courteous audiences. Interpreters translated the presentations made in English and fielded questions and replies. Nurses who attended this workshop demonstrated their curiosity from the outset. They asked questions, made comments, and continued discussions of content in the breaks, at meals, and in other social activities. The main objective of the workshop was to convene leaders of the major nursing associations in Ukraine to nurture the development of an All-Ukrainian Nursing Association. This association, founded three years earlier in 1997, had struggled to gain recognition and to attract members. At the same time, a number of specialty and regional nursing associations had been more successful in attracting members.

At issue was how to achieve some degree of unity among all of the Ukrainian nurses to enhance their ability to improve the professional capacity of nurses engaged in patient care. Developing a structure that would engage the existing specialty and regional nursing associations in initiatives of the country-wide association was viewed as a priority by the planners and participants. Curiosity about how the associations worked in the Ukraine and in the US was the equalizer for sharing among participants and faculty. The first lesson learned was that curiosity can lead to success. Openness to listen to each other contributed to the success of this workshop because everyone had some experience to share, and clearly the strength of Ukrainian nursing would be enhanced if the all-Ukrainian Nursing Association could build on the positive aspects of the regional and specialty Ukrainian nursing associations.

The second lesson learned was that nursing is universal. Presentations by presidents of the Operating Sisters Association in Moscow, the All-Russian Nurses Association, the Belarus Nurses Association, the Kiev Nursing Association, the All-Ukrainian Nursing Association, and the Psychiatric Nurses Association; by the Ministry of Health; and by the visiting faculty from the US were remarkably similar. Although it was evident that each association had unique aspects, all shared the commonality of working together to advance nursing science and to increase the capacity of nursing by working together for common causes to improve nursing practice and patient care. Availability of qualified nurses, staffing issues, educational needs, compensation, and nurse retention were examples of shared and common concerns. Most importantly, issues of having sufficient resources for patient care, keeping up-to-date in practice, and organizing nursing services to meet patient needs were priorities.

The will to create change was evident among the participants and facilitated the third lesson. Nurses who attended were eager to share their experiences and to learn. The level of energy and enthusiasm for the interactive learning, particularly the games played to demonstrate teamwork, were evidence of the engagement of attendees. The purpose of associations, the various ways they are structured, and the methods associations use to plan strategically and to achieve goals were generally accepted by the group. One of the greatest impediments to moving forward proved to be the commitment of time and energy as well as support from leaders external to healthcare organizations. The representative from the Ministry of Health was open about the ministry's support for nursing associations and the potential for mutual achievements.

Leaders of the existing nurses associations were committed to their associations' activities. The local unique healthcare institution's nursing service organization was viewed as both a catalyst and an impediment to strengthening the All-Ukrainian Nursing Association. Many participants perceived their own nursing service organizations to be the local equivalent of the All-Ukrainian Nursing Association. Awareness of the potential power of a country-wide association to improve patient care and nursing was enhanced in the interactive sessions. Developing the will to act, the intentionality of working toward a strong All-Ukrainian Nursing Association, made sense. Having the time in this workshop to meet and identify country-wide priorities was a critical first step in the change process, which strengthened the will to act intentionally.

The fourth important lesson learned from this workshop was that nursing throughout the world is viewed as a public service. Nursing practice is officially regulated in the country governance structure. This country-wide and regional governance of nursing is furthered at the institutional level where nursing is practiced. What nurses do for patients, their authority for practice, their autonomy in making decisions, and their ability to have a voice in creating and developing their environment for practice are priority questions raised at the workshop in the breakout sessions. These issues are common to nursing throughout the world. Nurses attending this workshop felt that their colleagues in specialty organizations needed to have more of a voice in local, regional, and national developments affecting nursing. They also felt that nurses should be intentionally included in the development of national plans for nursing and healthcare.

INTERACTIVE APPROACH TO LEARNING

Breakout sessions, games, discussion, and dialogue as well as informal conversations among participants at meal time and in breaks contributed to each participant's ability to engage in the workshop on a personal level. The formal presentations about associations provided the foundation for the interactive learning. For example, in breakout sessions and in games and informal conversation, participants discussed issues that impeded the growth of an all-Ukrainian nursing association. The workshop was planned to create an environment conducive to openness in sharing ideas and concerns. It was not only encouraged, but also expected that participants would voice these ideas and concerns openly. As a result, the strengths and weaknesses associated with diversity in nursing throughout the Ukraine and in specialty nursing practice could be discussed in a way that led to developing priorities for actions to build on strengths of diversity. Likewise, issues surrounding perceived divisiveness became a topic for discussion of ways to bring nursing together around priorities that all shared, while also recognizing and respecting the uniqueness of practice in various settings.

Nurses by nature of their work are concerned about patient safety, the quality of patient care, and the competence of nurses in practice. At this workshop, leader competencies were a focal topic. It was recognized that leaders provided mentoring, guidance, and authority for staff nurses. The initial brainstorming sessions focused on associations. Topics included creating and managing a country-wide association, engaging nurses in specialty and regional associations in a country-wide association, and bringing all of the associations together to effect change. Associations were viewed as a vehicle to accomplish goals for nursing. Leadership was viewed as essential to effecting change. The value of convening leaders for open dialogue, for action planning, and for working together toward a common good was demonstrated in this workshop. It was recognized that the critical mass of nurses in the country would have to be engaged to realize the goal of a country-wide association.

Lessons learned from this workshop include:

- Curiosity is an equalizer for diverse individuals and groups.

- Nursing is universal.

- The will to act to achieve results is essential.

- Nursing is a public service regulated by government.

Next steps related to what should happen to achieve the goal of a strong All-Ukrainian Nursing Association. Engaging the multitude of nurses in practice was viewed as one of the greatest challenges to achieve that goal. Many of the leaders who participated in this conference believed their first priority was to use the action learning methodology to work with their staff nurses. Developing professionally, keeping nurses up-to-date in their practice, and developing the will to act—or the intentionality to be an active part of a Ukrainian nursing association— were viewed as overwhelming but possible challenges by many leaders.

Program materials from this workshop were provided to each participant who could then use them with groups of nurses in their own local environments to share the learning. Content on teaching skills, curriculum development, meeting planning, and evaluation presented by association leaders conveyed two messages. The first message was that leaders are teachers. The second message was that associations can be helpful by providing education needed by all Ukrainian nurses using the notion of economy of scale. By participating in this workshop, each nurse leader was provided with skills to enhance performance in the local setting. In addition, each leader had the opportunity to develop a broader perspective of nursing in the Ukraine. The networking that occurred throughout the workshop was viewed by many as one of the most valuable and long-term benefits of the workshop.

THE OUTCOME

Workshop participants reached consensus about their next steps. They agreed to form a federation of associations in which each regional and specialty association would appoint a member to an advisory board that would meet regularly with the president of the All-Ukrainian Nursing Association to develop agendas relevant to nursing needs throughout the Ukraine. This federation model allowed each existing association to have individual members and to work on relevant activities. Rather than competing for members, these associations would be active in the All-Ukrainian Nursing Association, which would focus on advancing the profession as a whole and on improving health through collaboration among federation members and others. The All-Ukrainian Nursing Association would be responsible for developing country-wide nursing standards and guidelines, would be the official liaison with the Ministry of Health, and would be central in working with AIHA to continue the development of nursing leaders who would participate in the activities related to strengthening the All-Ukrainian Nursing Association and to developing its programs and services.

LESSONS LEARNED

This workshop was a professional encounter with nurses who shared common values, had common issues, and had a will to move forward to advance the profession. The lessons learned are valuable workshop outcomes that impact individual behaviors. They also serve as helpful concepts for those meeting with diverse groups or sharing their country experiences with others throughout the world. Be curious, for curiosity reduces impediments to learning; recognize and respect the universality of nursing; nurture the will to act, to improve; and appreciate the importance of nursing as a worldwide public service.

REFERENCES

Lawler, E. J., and Yoon, J. (1993). Power and the emergence of commitment behavior in negotiated exchange. *American Sociological Review, 58*(4), 465–481.

Lawler, E. J., and Yoon, J. (1996). Commitment in exchange relations: Test of theory of relational cohesion. *American Sociological Review, 61*, 89–108.

2

COLLABORATING FOR THE WORLD'S CHILDREN: COUNCIL OF INTERNATIONAL NEONATAL NURSES (COINN)

CAROLE KENNER, DNS, RNC, FAAN

ANITA FINKELMAN, MSN, RN

The Council of International Neonatal Nurses (COINN) evolved over a decade of informal communication among neonatal nurses globally. It started during Carole Kenner's presidency of the National Association of Neonatal Nurses (NANN) when she hosted what is now referred to as a meeting of 40 "close, global friends"—neonatal nursing leaders from around the world—in Seattle, Washington, during a neonatal conference. The reality was that few of us really knew each other, but we all shared a common bond—our desire to improve the outcomes for mothers and babies. The following year another neonatal nursing conference that incorporated international nursing as a theme was held in Washington, DC. A major outcome of this meeting was the commitment from neonatal nursing leaders from the United Kingdom (UK)—the oldest neonatal nursing group—Australia, New Zealand (NZ), and the United States (US) to hold an international neonatal nursing conference every three years. To date conferences have been held in Harrogate, England; Sydney, Australia; Toronto, Canada; and, in 2006, in Delhi, India.

With this humble beginning in 1994 of colleagues who wanted to discuss mutual concerns came the recognition of the need for a strong voice in neonatal nursing care at a global level. From that point to 2007 COINN has taken that dialogue to build an organization representing more than 50 countries and is on its way to being a fully incorporated 501 (c) 3–non-profit, tax exempt entity, which now has a partnership with the World Health Organization (WHO)'s Partnership for Maternal, Newborn, and Child Health (PMNCH) and affiliate status with the International Council of Nurses (ICN). How did COINN achieve such success so quickly?

DESCRIPTION OF PROJECT

Prior to the development of COINN no formal global effort of neonatal nurses existed to provide collaboration and assist one another in this complex area of healthcare. Why is it important to have a formal mechanism, such as a professional organization, that focuses on neonatal care? The problem of global infant mortality is staggering. A 2006 report from Save the Children estimates that globally about 2 million babies die within the first 24 hours of life and a total of 4 million babies die within the first month of life (Save the Children, 2007) Interventions do exist that can be implemented to prevent and treat many of the causes of infant mortality if an infrastructure can provide them, an infrastructure that is focused on the community, home-based, and considers critical cultural and communication needs of the community served. This infrastructure has to include nurses who are prepared to deliver the best care possible. The United Nations Millennium Development Goals (MDGs) include goals related to reducing infant mortality that must be reached if reducing child mortality and improving maternal health are ever to be accomplished.

COINN is one important approach that can assist in making a difference by using recognized global leaders in neonatal nursing care to:

1. Foster excellence in neonatal nursing

2. Promote the development of neonatal nursing as a recognized global specialty

3. Promote high standards of neonatal care

4. Enhance quality of care for our patients and families

5. Decrease health disparities

6. Improve healthcare outcomes.

The organization that needed to be created, COINN, emphasizes positive health outcomes for infants and families. COINN also acts as an international leader in the development and revision of professional standards of neonatal nursing. These activities, in turn, allow COINN to participate in international health policy work as experts in maternal and child health, most especially neonatal health to address problems described in these statistics (Save the Children, 2007):

- At present 38% of all child deaths globally occur during the neonatal period.

- One in every eight babies born in the US is premature according to the March of Dimes Birth Defects Foundation.

- On a global level, approximately 130 million infants are born annually; of these, 4 million die during the neonatal period (first 4 weeks of life).

The challenge for COINN was how to begin to meet these monumental and critical healthcare needs and mobilize the resources to respond in an organized manner. The first step with any global issue is to recognize that no one person or group can solve the problems; collaboration and partnership are required. COINN recognized from its focus groups over the past decade that many nurses in developing countries must do it all; no specialties exist, while other nurses are assigned to do neonatal care with little background. Nurses wanted COINN to find regional contacts to assist in these efforts with the idea that the regional contacts would be sensitive to cultural issues in that area of the world. In addition, using COINN's name and power would help raise the status of neonatal care in many countries. Initially, the emphasis was, and continues to be, on building capacity at country or local level. The ultimate outcome is providing nurses in developing countries with resources and skills to take on leadership and move care forward within their own countries.

As an organization, COINN has used a two-prong approach to increase its ability to collaborate with other nurses and to meet its goals. First, COINN initiated a membership effort directed at other healthcare professional organizations with common goals. This effort has been very successful and is ongoing.

- Australian College of Neonatal Nurses

- Canadian Association of Neonatal Nurses

- Danish Neonatal Nurses

- Finnish Neonatal Nurses

- New Zealand Association of Neonatal Nurses

- Scottish Neonatal Nurses Group

- Singapore Nurses Association—Pediatric and Neonatal Nurses

- South African Neonate, Infant, and Toddler Support Association

- Neonatal Network of Swedish Pediatric Nurses Association
- United Kingdom Neonatal Association
- National Association of Neonatal Nurses (NANN) (US)

The South African and Canadian associations of neonatal nurses have recently formed with the help of COINN.

Another unique feature of COINN is the development of regional access to address regional issues by neonatal experts who have an understanding of cultural and healthcare needs at the local level. Currently, COINN has representatives who serve as regional experts from Afghanistan, Argentina, Armenia, Australia, Botswana, Canada, Chile, Denmark, Ecuador, Estonia, Finland, Hong Kong, Hungary, Iceland, India, Iraq, Israel, Japan, Kenya, Korea, Kuwait, Lebanon, Liberia, Macedonia, Malaysia, Nepal, Netherlands, New Zealand, Nigeria, Norway, Pakistan, Peoples Republic of China, Portugal, Russia, Sao Tome, Scotland, Senegal, Singapore, South Africa, Swaziland, Sweden, Tanzania, Thailand, Turkey, United Arab Emirates, United Kingdom, United States, Uruguay, Vietnam, Zambia, and Zimbabwe.

The second major COINN initiative is directed at organizations and partnerships that COINN might join or build. The goal is to improve maternal and child healthcare by using global resources to work locally at the country level. This initiative will be ongoing as new relationships are developed. COINN has now partnered with the WHO Partnership for Safe Motherhood and Newborn Health and the UNICEF High-Level Global Leader meeting to engage in strategic planning and development of health policy that will improve neonatal care. COINN plans on expanding this type of initiative—building and strengthening collaborations.

OUTCOMES

The WHO Partnership organization has been in existence since 1999. At that time a steering committee of about 20 organizational representatives was created. This group included USAID, Save the Children, UNICEF, and others. The partnership's focus is to address the UN Millennium Development Goals. Three major tasks relate to this focus: (1) taking political action at grassroots (2) capacity building and (3) building regional networks. As a new organizational partner, COINN was asked to partner with FIGO (the International Federation of Gynecology and Obstetrics), the International Pediatric Association, and the International Confederation of Midwives. COINN's activities are centered on the continuum from preconception through adolescence. The four organizations who asked to work together envisioned their initial initiative to focus on position statements such as joint endorsements and standards and to examine areas of potential synergy. As the partnership has grown, it was suggested that we focus on the ICN's Girl Child Program, victimization, neonatal tetanus, infections, premature births, postpartum hemorrhage, and the use of skilled birth attendants, all of which related to the *Lancet* series "Neonatal Survival" (Lawn et al., 2005). In conjunction with this work, COINN was asked to participate in the UNICEF High-Level Global Leader meeting. This symposium on MDG 4, held in New York in September 2006, was co-organized by the government of Norway and UNICEF and co-chaired by the prime minister of Norway and the executive director of UNICEF. The MDG 4 goal "To reduce under-five mortality rate by two-thirds between 1990 and 2015" is an ambitious goal (UN, 2007). But, it can be achieved if we all work together and implement the most cost-effective and proven interventions at scale in countries with high rates of mortality and high numbers of child deaths. By focusing on this critical concern the symposium will indirectly help build momentum towards all the MDGs and the Millennium Declaration.

In addition to these initiatives, COINN is assisting Kenya, Russia, and Tanzania to form neonatal nursing groups. In Zimbabwe a land-reform program has affected women by placing them in remote areas without road or telephone networks, so they cannot access antenatal clinical services. COINN is helping to address this and other critical issues such as poor maternal nutrition that leads to poor neonatal outcomes. COINN is working to develop a pilot study to determine the best interventions to use and to empower the nursing mother with money-generating products so they can sustain themselves. A link with Kenyan and South African regional contacts has helped with this endeavor. In Iraq the on-ground nurses are requesting assistance with standards of care and with the setting up of an exchange program for Iraqi nurses to come to the University of Oklahoma for a 3–6 month period of study.

UNEXPECTED CHALLENGES AND OPPORTUNITIES

The main challenge is to obtain funding for the many potential projects. Most of the countries requesting assistance are in no position to pay for any services. As a non-profit organization with an international focus, COINN has raised more red flags in its journey to full corporate status because of the political scrutiny of tax-exempt, international organizations. Many companies that either act as sponsors or have grant foundations are available to COINN, yet they do not want to invest until there is a track record, something hard to obtain without funds. The other main challenges are not to overcommit the few resources we have and to be ethical about what we can and cannot do in a certain time period.

The opportunities for neonatal nursing collaboration are expansive. Having obtained a place in the WHO community, having gained affiliate status with ICN, and having been an invited participant as the only nursing organization at the UNICEF High-Level Global Leader meeting, COINN has already made an impact. COINN continues to receive requests from other countries and organizations to address the maternal and child health healthcare needs.

LESSONS LEARNED

The lessons that we have learned are that you cannot be all things to all people and countries. The needs are vast, and the organization can quickly feel overwhelmed. It also takes a lot of time and energy and perseverance to get an organization firmly established. If we had it to do over again, we would have informally organized for a longer time before committing to a formal, corporate structure with associated costs.

WORDS OF WISDOM TO OTHERS DOING INTERNATIONAL WORK

International work requires a passion. It is a group effort—an organization's expertise coupled with the knowledge of the country requesting the partnership. Too often international partners try to impose values on each other. This does not work. The work is like a marriage with give and take and with an understanding of each other's strengths and weaknesses. Trust is built on relationships, and relationships take time. Do not be in a rush to "save the world." Do it one step at a time.

REFERENCES

Lawn, J. E., Cousens, S., and Zupan, J., for the Lancet Neonatal Survival Steering Team. (2005). Neonatal survival 1: 4 million neonatal deaths: when? where? why? Retrieved on 3 October 2007 from http://www.who.int/child-adolescent-health/publications/NEONA-TAL/Lancet_NSS.htm

Save the Children (2007).. Retrieved on February 26, 2007, from http://www.savethechildren.org/newsroom/2006/first-24-hours-of-life-most-dangerous.html

United Nations (2007). UN Millennium Development Goals. Retrieved on February 26, 2007, from http://www.un.org/millenniumgoals/

3

WAR IS NOTHING LIKE YOU THINK. IT'S MUCH MORE!

LEAH CURTIN, RN, MS, MA, FAAN

The Franciscan Sisters of the Poor Health System, under a grant from the American International Health Alliance (AIHA), agreed to become partners with hospitals in parts of war-torn Yugoslavia, most notably Croatia, even though the hostilities were not quite at an end. Health-care personnel made exchange visits, and everyone learned a great deal. However, Michael Hoffman, chief executive officer (CEO) of the Franciscan Sisters of the Poor Health Foundation and Sr. Joanne Schuster, president of the Franciscan Sisters of the Poor Health System, were concerned about what might happen to these hospitals when the partnership came to an end. They were operating on a shoestring. Their only source of funds was the government, and the government had many other problems and obligations. Thus, the hospitals frequently were simply not sent operating costs. They had no other source of funds and often found themselves in desperate straits. They were so desperate that personnel often worked for months without pay.

In light of this concern, Sr. Joanne traveled to Croatia to teach administrative teams at the hospitals in Zadar and Biograd how to create a foundation and raise the money needed to underwrite care. A book to be sold in the United States (US) was part of this effort. I had met Sr. Joanne while doing some consultation for the Franciscan Sisters of the Poor Health System. She knew that I was an editor and writer, so she asked me if I would be willing to research and write a book, all of the proceeds of which would be donated to a special fund devoted to helping restore and rehabilitate children injured in the war. I would determine the approach, scope, and content of the book in consultation with Sr. Joanne and Michael Hoffman. I was fascinated by the project, so I agreed to accompany Sr. Joanne on a trip to Zadar, Croatia, in 1999, where she introduced me to health care leaders in Zadar and Biograd. They did not really understand the project, but they opened doors and provided access. Most importantly, they assigned Patricjia Padelin, child psychologist at the hospital in Zadar, to help me.

Priya Chandra, AIHA's country coordinator for Croatia, provided invaluable support, arranged meetings, and facilitated the research and communication essential for verisimilitude. A Croatian-born child psychiatrist currently living in the US, Maria Krocker-Tuskan, reviewed the manuscript, discussed Croatian history with me, and corrected errors arising from difficulties with translation and, occasionally, cultural misunderstandings.

Setting the Course

As I began preparing to write the book, I tried to learn as much as I could about the impact of war on children. According to UNICEF, the ratio of soldiers to civilians wounded or killed in armed conflicts during the 20th century has reversed itself. In World War I one civilian was killed or wounded for every nine soldiers, while in today's conflicts, nine civilian casualties occur for each military one (Zivcic, 1993). About 60% of civilian casualties are children. Social workers and psychologists described their traumas: loss of family members, especially one or both parents; loss of parental support and protection; loss of home and family living; malnutrition; incarceration, sometimes in detention camps but usually in attempts to keep them from harm; loss of personal space; loss of physical abilities if the child was wounded; loss of a sense of security and stability; loss of innocence (a näive belief that others will not harm you); loss of educational opportunities and school life; the problems associated with living in an extremely poor environment with stressed adults, and exposure to horrors beyond imagining (Ajdukovic, 1998).

Yet, the unspeakable horrors of war are themselves almost cleansed of their horror when analyzed and objectified. As appalling as the statistics are to read, they only describe reality; they don't reveal it. Traveling into the war zone revealed it. The utter devastation is stunning. Pockmarks in ruined buildings give mute testimony to the violence; barely one square foot remains undamaged. Most of the roads had craters surrounded by the stereotypical marks of rockets and mortars and bombs. School buildings, apartments, homes, and many shops are rubble.

How do the children themselves perceive these experiences? I wondered. Perhaps the work of artist Emil Robert Tanay comes closest to capturing them. Tanay and his colleagues worked with refugee children in Zagreb, and Tanay in particular worked with children under siege in Mostar. His work? To help children express their experiences through drawings. The children were not told to paint pictures of what they were seeing, but rather of what they were feeling. They also were encouraged to depict scenes from their lives before the war. Most of the children's paintings used visual metaphors to express their fears and seek comfort; in some they used color to express the sensations, even the smell of war.

I decided to use both the visual expression of the experiences of the children of the Balkan conflict and their own words to help people understand the reality of war. The book would be unique in the sense that the stories are told from a child's point of view. I would gather the children's stories and recollections in interviews with them and their families, in dialogue with professional colleagues, and through review of the relevant literature. I could collect the children's art simply by asking the children I interviewed to paint a picture for me. As it turned out, I also collected artwork from others: Patricija Padelin, and Suncokret, a voluntary Croatian refugee organization located in Zagreb. After short exposure to the politics, violence, and instability of the Balkans and after taking into account the fact that Slobodan Milosavic was still in power, I decided to fictionalize the stories I collected to protect the children's identities, while nonetheless protecting the integrity of the their experiences. Now, I thought, all that needed to be done was to collect the stories, the artwork, and write. I was wrong, of course!

LESSONS TO LEARN BEFORE STARTING

The first thing I had to do was to win Patricija Padelin's trust, and then the trust of my translators, the children, and their parents. Patricija didn't trust me because so many people had come to Croatia to exploit the war for personal gain. "People want to come and see these children, especially the ones who were wounded. We're supposed to display them for a few kuna (Croatian currency) to journalists from Germany, England, France, and the US—as if they were freaks in a carnival."

Indeed, physicians introduced me to the first child, who I later learned from Patrijia was told to disrobe in front of me and display his amputated limb and other scars. His aunt stayed to enforce the discipline (both of his parents had been killed in the war). He was so embarrassed and humiliated that he would not even look at me, much less talk to me or draw pictures for me. Clearly the purpose of my project was not understood, and it took time and patient persistence to get this across. Patricija Padelin is a child psychologist who worked with the children of Zadar before, during, and after the war. She understands their problems, and she walks through their fears with them because she shared them herself. "I was scared like a rabbit," she says. "I shook with fear." Because she stayed with them throughout all their tribulations, she is trusted. They know she understands. So, once I won Patricija's trust, parents, children, teachers, and health professionals all seemed willing to help. Some even demanded to do so!

The next thing was to learn to understand the culture, the people, and their history. I believe that you cannot understand a people unless you understand their history and culture. For this reason, I always visit museums when I am traveling, and I try to learn about the people through their history. You can also learn a great deal about a people if you explore their myths, religions, and the stories they tell their children. Patricija took me to museums, and she collected children's fairy tales and stories for me to read (she had to translate).

Then came the need to understand acts of war and how people react in war. Darija, 13 years old and living just outside the town of Biograd, told me, "War is nothing like I thought it would be. Not like on television, not like in books, not like anything you could even begin to imagine. It is to be so afraid that you cannot sleep even when there are no bombs. It is to see everything, *everything*, destroyed. I cannot speak of those who are dead, my heart is still in bandages. I am happy I am still alive, but I am ashamed too." Neven, who at 19 spoke 7 languages, was my translator on two of my visits. Neven spent most of the war in Zadar and the rest as a refugee in Rome. He stoically translated Darija's words and later added some of his own. He told me tales of the bombings and of collecting shells (only some of them spent) in the streets around his home, of hauling drinking water from trucks, of protecting churches and historic buildings with sandbags, and of sewer systems that no longer work.

Finally, I had to learn how to listen and learn from the listening. I had to listen without judging and without reacting, no matter how hard it was to listen to what people were telling me.

The children told me of the smell of war: a combination of chordite, cement and plaster dust, burning materials, and even people, sewerage, sweat, and fear. They told me what it's like, that it doesn't hurt much at first when you are wounded, and how the children handled what they saw and heard. "I could not look anymore, and I would not let the younger children look either. We hid and kept very quiet. We tried to keep even from hearing, but we could not. They must have done this [torture] to each one of the old people; some of them laughed and said coarse words. All the while the old ones screamed and cried and begged for death. And then, when they were done with that, we heard the guns again. They murdered them. We did not move or even hardly breathe, not for a long time after they left. We do not speak of the time we were on our own or of what we did and what we saw. Unless someone asks. You asked."

One thing I learned: one may learn to understand how people react in war situations, but there is no reasonable explanation for "war crimes." There is no understanding them, and there is no way possible to exact justice for them. It may be possible to forgive them, but in my darker moments, I cannot see how.

Writing, Reviewing, and Publishing

I also learned that I must deal with myself. Many of the children's stories were too much for me to bear. At times I *needed* to go home. I needed not to know anymore. It was a lesson put sorely to the test as later, at home, I reviewed my notes and began to write. To write a story well, you have to enter into the experiences of your characters, to experience what they are experiencing, to feel what they are feeling. Many times I could not write anymore because I was crying. Many times I had to force myself back to the computer. And then I had to subject what I had written to a Croatian-born child psychiatrist for correction and review. The finest compliment I have ever received is when she said, "I think you have actually caught the children's experiences."

Perhaps the worst thing for me personally was to experience some of their losses firsthand. In the midst of my writing, I received a packet from Patricija. When I opened it, I was delighted to find 52 pictures drawn by the children of Skabrnje, many of whom I had met and interviewed, and I found a note. Patricija had visited the village and talked with many of the children at the school. She asked them for the pictures and for stories about themselves and what they will "be" when they grow up for the lady from America. When I saw their pictures, my heart lifted. Then I noticed a penciled note from Patricija. Written in haste on the piece of cardboard she'd inserted to protect the pictures from injury, it was barely legible. She wrote:

Dear Leah,

I have collected these pictures for you from the chidren recently returned to Skabrnje. But, in the two weeks since they drew them, three have been killed by land mines.

Patricija

As the project neared completion, I had to choose a name. I selected *Sunflowers in the Sand.* The word *sunflower* in the Croatian language also means "turning toward the sun." Children instinctively turn toward the light; even a little bit of light will do. The sunflower's roots, however, must be firmly planted in the ground for it to grow to its full height. Today's children—not just the children of the Balkans, but all children—have their roots sunk into the shifting sands of adult politics, adult greed, and far too often, adult cruelty. That is why I added the subtitle: *Stories from the Children of War.*

MEASURES OF SUCCESS

The purpose of this project was to demonstrate to people from another culture and economic system (communism) how to raise money to help cover the costs of care in hospitals. As part of the overall effort, which was a success, the book project also was successful. To date, the sale of *Sunflowers in the Sand: Stories from the Children of War* has raised tens of thousands of dollars, and it is still selling. The book also was reviewed in the New York Times' *Sunday Book Section,* the gold standard for authors; barely one in a thousand published books is chosen for review in the *Times,* and one of the children's pictures was run with the story.

LESSONS LEARNED

What words of wisdom could I offer those who choose to work in another culture? Well, this was neither my first, nor my last opportunity to do so, but what I have to say seems trite. First, do not judge the culture. Learn about it. Visit the museums. Read the fairytales. Learn the myths. Learn at least how to say "hello," "goodbye," and "thank you." If you are going to stay for any period of time, learn the language. Even then, do not undertake any meaningful work without a translator at your side. Be open to suggestions and ask for help. Check and double-check to make sure that people actually *do* understand you and are not simply being polite. Do not think that everything you have to offer will be needed, wanted, or accepted. A little humility goes a long way toward gaining acceptance. Do not talk about yourself or how things are done in the US unless you are specifically asked to do so, and then, be brief. Learn about how things are done in the country and culture in which you are working, and do not make comparisons (particularly negative ones) to the US. The country you are visiting is not, never will be, and should not be the US. Learn to appreciate the similarities as well as the differences. Keep your opinions to yourself, and you will learn a lot more than you ever dreamed you could.

REFERENCES

Ajdukovic, M. and Ajdukovic, D, (1993). Psychological well-being of refugee children. *Child Abuse & Neglect,* 17(6), 843-54.

Zivcic, Ivanka. (1993). "Emotional reactions of children to war stress in Croatia." *Journal of the American Academy of Child & Adolescent Psychiatry*, 32(4), July, 709.

4

PROCESS IMPROVEMENTS IN GLOBAL HEALTH

PAMELA AUSTIN THOMPSON, MS, RN, FAAN

Process is about how and why we do things to accomplish specific goals. It is a map for getting from one place to another. In the United State (US), "quality improvement" is a well-known process that encompasses significant tools and methodologies. It enjoys both popularity and disfavor, but for most acute care settings such as hospitals, it has become a thread in the fabric of the internal operations. It is one of the ways that we improve what we are doing and that we introduce change to our dynamic systems of care.

In the 1990s, I was involved with an international project that partnered an academic medical center in the US with three hospitals in Zagreb, Croatia. The project began when Croatia was still involved in the war that engulfed the Balkans in the 1990s, a conflict between Bosnia-Herzegovina, Serbia, and Croatia. Croatia had recently declared independence from Yugoslavia. The country was a new republic, and it was eager to create new infrastructures, especially for healthcare. Our project became a small part of this work to build a new country.

I served the project as leader of the administration and nursing initiatives. The project had a detailed 3-year work plan that outlined how each aspect of the partnership would further the goals of the three hospitals for specific administrative and clinical programs. Central to the entire plan was a belief on the part of the U.S. partners that quality improvement was the foundation teaching for all of the initiatives. We believed that if our partners understood and could practice these concepts, they would be equipped to address future projects on their own. We had no idea how critical this initial assumption was to become.

PROJECT DESCRIPTION

The U.S. team developed a 10-day educational program that taught the concepts of quality improvement and process redesign to the project leaders in each hospital. The venue for the 10 days was away from the hospital at a retreat setting. Three separate sessions for three groups of leaders were conducted over the three years. Each group consisted of a 35-member interdisciplinary team consisted of nurses, physicians, and administrators from the three hospitals. The curriculum was designed to include significant experiential learning and leadership development. Content included the basics of quality improvement methodologies, techniques, and tools such as process charting, brainstorming, affinity grouping, meeting management, and statistical analysis. It also included content for situational leadership, collaboration, teamwork, project planning, and creativity. Didactic content was blended with games and activities, which were novel methodologies for the participants. During these introductory sessions, the individual projects were developed that became the vehicles for ongoing learning and change.

The U.S. leaders assisted the hospital teams with their project designs and action plans. Two examples of the projects developed include 1) developing a family visitation program in a pediatric infectious disease hospital and 2) developing a collaborative practice model for an inpatient cardiology unit. In both examples, the Croatian teams outlined their plans and designs based on the process design work that they had done in the initial sessions. Every effort was made to link the process of improvement to their expressed outcomes. The Croatian work teams were responsible for identifying what needed to change in their system and the final characteristics of success.

OUTCOMES ACHIEVED

In both of the preceding examples, the groups achieved their desired outcomes. However, they learned as much in the process of doing the work as in the final project accomplishment. The project outlines guided their work, and they stayed focused on "what do we want this to look like in the end, what will success look like." The focus on the end result encouraged mid-project course corrections as the projects took shape and the unexpected occurred. It provided an easy way to change the process when it wasn't working, to introduce new ideas, and to solidify processes when they did work. In the end, the family visiting hours were implemented, and the milieu of the cardiology unit was grounded in collaborative practice principles—individual journeys that are stories in themselves.

UNEXPECTED OUTCOMES AND CHALLENGES

The most obvious challenge was translating a U.S. process for use in a Croatian system with unique characteristics. The Croatian work environment had been somewhat regimented, hierarchical, and rules-based, but that was changing rapidly. The forming of the new government and the impact of the war had created significant ambiguity and turmoil. There was significant stress on what had been a stable environment. Group process decision making had not been the norm, and all of the tools and techniques introduced for the quality improvement processes were new. Interestingly, however, many of these challenges turned out to be positive factors in many ways. The participants were eager for change, and even though the process of change caused the usual discomfort, they had a greater willingness to embrace new ideas and a lack of preconceived resistance.

Another added benefit was the professional relationship between physicians and nurses, which was congenial and positive. Although rigid professional boundaries existed between them, their interpersonal relationships created strong teamwork and collaboration among the project groups.

LESSONS LEARNED

The most important lesson learned came as feedback from one of the participants. He told us that we didn't just teach him how to implement a specific project; we taught him how to "think" differently about the work. That turned out to be a sustainable change because the processes that they had learned were applicable and adaptable to a multitude of future projects. We also learned to listen to the assessments that our partners made regarding how to change and what to change. They knew the strengths and barriers in their systems far better than anyone from the outside did. Our role turned out to be more coaching, mentoring, investing in, and trusting our partners to design the strategies based on their knowledge of the systems. This empowered the Croatian team to embrace the design and to take ownership of the processes.

WORDS OF WISDOM

It is important to remember that a process that is successful in the US isn't automatically going to be successful in an international arena. Teaching a process like quality improvement can work very well if the individuals using it can adapt it as necessary to their culture and environment. The process becomes the framework for projects that are designed to address the specific situations of an environment. This process of adaptation creates a better fit and positions projects for ownership by those doing the implementation.

It is inadvisable to take a specific U.S. project plan and think that it can be implemented exactly the same way in another environment. This also does not teach a process as much as it teaches the specific tasks of a project. This learning is not as transferable as process learning. As the participant told me, you have to learn to think differently, and then you can apply that learning and thinking to any future project. Process is how and why we do things. Teaching process concepts so that others can add the "what needs to be done to accomplish the goals" can be a successful strategy for working with international partners. It is built on a mutual respect for who brings what expertise to the table and creates the potential for mutual benefit to both parties.

5

Nursing as an International Relationship

Kathleen A. Bower, DNSc, RN, FAAN

Background

Nursing is, in large part, based on relationships—with patients and families, healthcare team members and colleagues. As a result, national and international networks are created both deliberately and spontaneously. Because an enthusiasm for sharing knowledge exists, opportunities for collaboration abound. I have had the privilege of working with colleagues throughout the world, from Canada to Australia, Singapore, Japan, South Africa, Dubai, Spain, Great Britain, and many other locations. Most of the international experiences I have enjoyed are related to the work that I and others did at New England Medical Center in Boston in inventing and implementing clinical paths and provider-based case management. Here, I highlight two international experiences.

Project Description—Barcelona, Spain

I have had the privilege of working with the Santa Madrona Nursing School in Barcelona, Spain, for more than 10 years, an opportunity created by networking. A U.S. colleague and previous client taught a nursing management module in the school's master's program for a number of years. The director of the school was (and is) acutely aware of new trends in healthcare in the US and was interested in providing information about clinical paths and case management to her students as well as to the area healthcare community. Through this connection, I was invited to teach a workshop on those topics for local hospitals and to provide 3 days of classes for the students; I readily agreed.

I arrived at the school on the first day of the master's course that I was teaching, more than a bit jet-lagged and a bit disoriented. I would be working through a simultaneous translator, which created some trepidation for me because it would change the amount of material that I could teach as well as my pacing. Fortunately, my colleague was there, providing a helpful bridge to the school and its students.

In reality, the 3 days went well. The simultaneous translator was excellent and a great resource. The students were a delight to teach, interested, willing to describe their environments and issues, and eager to learn new approaches to dealing with their situations. They were, however, quick to identify where the U.S. healthcare experience differed from that in Barcelona and how those differences created the need to change some of the approaches I was recommending and teaching. It was a tremendous learning experience for me. It reaffirmed for me that issues of health are similar throughout the world, particularly in nations where basic survival is not the key problem of life. It also taught me that healthcare issues can be discussed, even through a simultaneous translator.

It has been more than 10 years since that first experience with healthcare in Barcelona. I have taught at the school each year since that introduction with the same experience—great students, great translator, tremendous learning, and a profound appreciation for the work that my Spanish colleagues are undertaking. Over the past few years, I have had students talk with me about the work they have been doing in their own organizations. It is a delight to see that they have implemented clinical paths and can articulate their results, and they attribute it to the material that I taught in previous years. One recent workshop participant has worked with her organization to create case management in the ambulatory care system with positive outcomes, a tribute to her and the administrative team at her organization.

PROJECT DESCRIPTION—SINGAPORE

Singapore is an example of a country grappling with an increase in elderly and chronically ill citizens while simultaneously attempting to manage healthcare costs. My experience with the Singapore healthcare system began with an e-mail from a member of the Ministry of Health requesting a meeting during a U.S. trip with the goal of learning more about clinical paths and case management. This request was accommodated, and we spent a few hours talking about the origin of clinical paths and case management, including potential outcomes, issues, barriers, and required resources. He had done research via the Internet on these topics and seemed to feel that these care management strategies would be very useful in Singapore.

Clinical paths appeared to be the first order of interest for the Ministry. In general, I have found case management to be a bit more confusing to clinicians in other countries; they cannot make the immediate translation to their own situations as easily as they can with clinical paths.

I believe that is because case management, as we have practiced it in the United States (US) and as it is seen in the literature, has a greater financial focus than clinicians in many countries have assumed. I have learned that, rather than focusing on the financial aspects of case management, an emphasis on coordinating care for highly complex individuals resonates with clinicians; it seems that complexity is experienced worldwide.

After that visit in the US, I was invited to present at a Pan-Pacific conference being hosted by the Ministry of Health and several hospitals in Singapore. This was followed by consultation at interested individual hospitals. I found much interest during the conference and the individual hospital consultation. The participants were clearly analyzing the information within the context of their healthcare situations.

Subsequent to that first experience in Singapore, I was invited to be a Visiting Expert for the Ministry of Health (MOH) with a focus on clinical paths. This was quite an honor as I would be the first nurse so designated by the MOH. The format was again a conference followed by time with individual hospitals. This time, however, the consultation visits with the individual hospitals was at a much higher level. There clearly had been attempts (many successful) at implementing clinical paths, and the discussions were more focused on highlighting what had been done with a request for analysis and recommendations for ongoing implementation. These were robust discussions with individuals who now had experience in using clinical paths.

In the years that have followed, I have watched as clinicians from Singapore, many whose names I recognize, have presented papers and lectures at conferences throughout the world. It is an honor to know that I launched the knowledge of those presenters.

Lessons Learned

- Healthcare needs and issues of individuals and populations are similar throughout the world. Culture and politics influence how those needs are met and issues are addressed. But the core is remarkably consistent throughout most of the world. Of course, in some corners of the world healthcare is a daily struggle, one that clinicians and others sometimes lose.

- The aging population, expanding numbers of individuals with chronic illnesses, and paying for increasing healthcare costs are universal concerns.

- The role of nursing in other countries may differ from that in the US. This is the result of politics, regulations, supply and demand, and other factors. It is important to explore nuances in nursing's role as it exists in the host country while formulating a response or opinion.

- Techniques for treating many illnesses are likely to be similar throughout many parts of the world. However, the impetus for managing that care and how care is organized may be very different from that in the US. Again, it is important to understand resources, priorities, and politics when making recommendations. I have encouraged many nurses to become politically active, particularly when they articulate needs of citizens and patients that are going unmet. For many, this is an idea that is difficult to consider.

- Ask questions and get lots of additional information before expressing an opinion if possible. Information about the local issues and processes provides a better context for your response.

- Practitioners in every country have great pride in the care they provide—and rightly so. A key to success in other countries is to have and reflect a great deal of respect for the skill and knowledge of colleagues in those countries.

- The Internet has created a worldwide healthcare community. We can discuss healthcare situations and strategies with individuals throughout the world with the click of a computer key. That technology also enables clinicians who are invited to work with colleagues in other countries to learn more about the culture of healthcare before they leave home.

- Some words and phrases are perfectly acceptable to Americans but are highly insulting to colleagues in other cultures. Sometimes uncovering what those words and phrases are involves experiential learning, and a great deal of apologizing and back-pedaling.

- Humor (particularly joking) does not translate well. Use it sparingly and watch the reaction of the audience very carefully. If possible, use a host colleague as a sounding board.

- Compassion, sincerity, enthusiasm for the care of individuals, generosity with knowledge, curiosity, respect, and enjoyment of colleagues does translate very well. Tone of voice, expression, and body language transcend oral language.

- Be curious, very curious. Colleagues in other cultures have a great deal of knowledge and many, many great ideas about how to deal with health related issues. You will learn as much as you teach—sometimes more.

- Time has different meaning in different parts of the world. In some countries, promptness is important. In others, promptness is not firmly embedded as a concept. It is up to the guest to figure it out and go with the flow by being prompt if that is the expectation and being flexible if promptness is not a local virtue.

- Bring a small gift to your hosts, particularly one that has meaning or represents where you live.

- Know that preparation time for hosts and host organizations is likely to be longer than expected, particularly if material must be translated. It is particularly important (and respectful) to provide information and materials in a timely manner.

- Safety is an important concern, particularly when traveling to more exotic or distant parts of the world.

  - Know where the American embassy is and how to contact it.

  - Explore the accommodations where you will staying and make sure that it appears safe to you. If not, negotiate a different setting.

  - Determine how you will get from the airport to your accommodations, particularly if you will be arriving late at night.

- Do not hesitate to accept the opportunity to work with colleagues in other countries. It is an enriching experience that provides many positive memories, even if it is not highly rewarding financially.

6

THE CHINA EXPERIENCE

BEVERLY J. McELMURRY, RN, EdD, FAAN

China's AIDS epidemic continues to grow, with an estimated 70,000 new HIV infections in 2005. The latest data indicate that 650,000 (range 390,000 to 1,100,000) people are now living with HIV in China and that overall HIV prevalence is now estimated at approximately 0.05 percent (UNAIDS, 2005).

As in most regions of the world, nurses in China are at the forefront of health care, and there aren't enough nurses to meet communities' needs. This is particularly problematic in provinces with populations vulnerable to HIV, including injecting drug users and sex workers. Many nurses have not had access to training that would equip them to confront an epidemic that is fueled by poverty, lack of education, and gender inequality. Some of the challenges China faces concerning HIV/AIDS are related to the fears, attitudes, and beliefs of both lay persons and health professionals. Other challenges arise because of insufficient managerial and administrative expertise needed for comprehensive HIV/AIDS care, prevention, and treatment, including anti-retroviral (ARV) therapy.

In recent years, progress has been made in nursing development, including education and service. However, nursing in China still faces multiple and critical challenges. These include caring for an aging population, rising non-communicable disease rates, and a changing health system that is struggling to provide equitable curative and community-based care in an era of rapid demographic changes and diminished resources. The advent of HIV/AIDS has compounded the existing challenges to nursing. Consequently, the China Nurses' Leadership Initiative for HIV/AIDS Care and Prevention program (Carol Christiansen, RN, PhD, director) was developed through a collaborative effort to assist nurses in their efforts to mitigate the impact of HIV/AIDS. This program is housed at the University of Illinois at Chicago WHO Collaborating Center for International Primary Health Care (PHC) Development.

DESCRIPTION OF PROJECT

PARTNERS

This ongoing project involves multiple collaborators, allowing for the highest possible levels of cooperation, local involvement, and sustainability. Partners and lead personnel include the University of Illinois at Chicago College of Nursing (Carol Christiansen), World Health Organization (WHO) (Kathleen Fritsch), Maryknoll China Service Project/Hong Kong (Scott Harris, MD), Catholic Medical Mission Board (Barbara Smith), Chinese Nurses Association/Beijing (Huaping Liu), and the Nursing Division of the Ministry of Health/Beijing (Yanhoung Guo). The initiative is accomplished by fostering collaborative working relationships and networks between academic institutions, central and provincial nursing associations, and health ministries.

Key principles guiding the strategic directions of the program are (1) partnership and collaboration to provide mutual support focused on common goals, (2) relevance to ensure that the project is guided by China's health needs, (3) ownership to promote local involvement, full participation, and nursing leadership development, and (4) ethical action to ensure that project objectives and service provision are based on equity and accessibility. Both HIV prevention and patient care largely depend on an educated public, health workforce development, health program infrastructure development, and HIV/AIDS-related policy initiatives.

From 2003 through 2006, international and national partners developed and tested a comprehensive HIV/AIDS curriculum and followed up with multiple provincial training workshops. The program was implemented in partnership with key universities in provinces with high HIV prevalence rates. During this time period, 745 nurses were trained and nursing faculty from Xian Jiaotong (Xiaomei Li, RN, MS) and Sichuan Universities (Xiaolian Jiang, RN, PhD) were prepared as nurse trainers in preparation for future work.

PROGRAM

The aim of the China Nurses' Leadership Initiative for HIV/AIDS Care and Prevention is to assist in strengthening capacity in HIV/AIDS-related knowledge and skills for nurses working in clinical and public health practice in high-impact provinces. During 2005–2006, this was accomplished in Yunnan, Guangxi, Anhui, and Xinjiang provinces by focusing on two key activities: (1) the introduction of a 5-day interactive HIV/AIDS training program and (2) the provision of a culturally relevant and comprehensive HIV/AIDS curriculum with supporting educational materials in chronic and palliative care. The presence, skills, knowledge, and sensitivity of the more than 1.3 million nurses in China are of critical importance in the response to HIV/AIDS as they can affect not only the health of their patients, but also the attitudes and awareness of the general publication.

PROCESS

Assessments in specific provinces enabled lead personnel to meet with Chinese Non Governmental Organizations (NGOs), various agency representatives, and nursing leaders. As a project map emerged, it was evident that a multifaceted program was required, including the provision of trainers with expertise in HIV/AIDS, plans for health professional education and training, and culturally relevant and appropriate curriculum development.

TRAINING

Each session included time for feedback on content and pre- and post-testing for evaluative purposes, as well as educational reviews and/or training on opportunistic infections, behavior and gender issues, prevention, community planning, mobilization, the role of social service agencies and NGOs, and the epidemiology of HIV/AIDS—transmission, immune responses, progression, and testing methods. The role of IV drug use, blood exchange, commercial sex, poverty, support for caregivers, home-based care, nutrition, counseling, terminal and palliative care, and other psychosocial issues was also addressed. Evening Q&A sessions were also made available, and were well attended.

Educational materials were developed for the training of trainers, with an aim to replicate the model within China. Nurses are prepared for practice and teaching with specialized training in the areas of women's health in China, mother-to-child (MTC) transmission, ethical issues and the stigma surrounding HIV/AIDS, nurse-managed care, community assessment, and identification of vulnerable populations.

Many provinces have requested copies of the HIV/AIDS curriculum for use in nursing schools. Modules highlighted by students as most useful, include counseling, HIV/AIDS basic knowledge, community care and palliative care, clinical care, and universal precautions/occupational safety. This last topic was one of the most popular in the course. Nurses openly stated their fears and prejudices about caring for someone known to be, or perceived to be, HIV positive. Most nurses stated they did not know how to protect themselves in the workplace and were unsure of the principles underlying universal precautions. This has promoted fear and increased the stigma and discrimination. Nurses voiced concerns about self-care and transmission prevention in resource-poor areas where gloves, masks, and goggles are not widely available. The universal precautions and occupational safety session also included information about post-exposure prophylaxis (PEP).

With regard to demographics, most of the participants were older, with a number of years of working experience. With the exception of Anhui province, the majority were also actively caring for patients and families affected by HIV/AIDS. This helps in understanding their expressed interests in clinical care, occupational exposure, palliative care, and counseling. The fact that many nurses came from positions with management responsibilities implies that they will have opportunities to educate staff and influence policy development in their places of employment.

OUTCOMES

The evaluation data for the training activities in Guangxi, Yunnan, Anhui, and Xinjiang provinces is qualitative, quantitative, and observational. The key objective in the program was the completion of training for 500 nurses in essential HIV/AIDS knowledge and skills by August of 2006 in those four provinces. This target objective was exceeded; a total of 682 nurses were trained (Yunnan—136; Guangxi—135; Anhui—155; and, Xinjiang—250).

Outputs associated with this key objective included the formation of provincial management teams to plan and support trainings, development of culturally sensitive training materials, and monitoring and evaluation. Indicators of goal achievement included the number of trained personnel and the reporting of pre- and post-testing. Each of the four provinces saw statistically significant score gains in HIV/AIDS knowledge, attitudes, and understanding as demonstrated between the pre- and post-tests. (See Tables C-6.1, C-6.2, and C-6.3.)

TABLE C-6.1. PROVINCIAL AND OVERALL PRE- AND POST-TEST ANALYSIS OF CHINESE NURSE PARTICIPANTS KNOWLEDGE OF HIV/AIDS PREVENTION, TRANSMISSION, TREATMENT, AND NURSING CARE, 2006 (N = 643).

| Province | Mean Score | | Score Gain | Statistically Significant p Value |
	Pre-Test	Post-Test		
Yunnan	12.85	15.87	+3.02	$p < 0.001$
Guangxi	13.15	15.62	+2.47	$p < 0.001$
Anhui	13.47	15.28	+1.81	$p < 0.001$
Xinjiang	13.39	15.29	+1.9	$p < 0.001$
Overall	13.19	15.48	+2.29	$p < 0.001$

TABLE C-6.2. PROVINCIAL AND OVERALL PRE- AND POST-TEST ANALYSIS OF HIV/AIDS ATTITUDES OF CHINESE NURSES, 2006 (N = 643).

| Province | Mean Score | | Score Gain | Statistically Significant p Value |
	Pre-Test	Post-Test		
Yunnan	19.74	32.60	+12.86	$p < 0.001$
Guangxi	20.33	36.17	+15.84	$p < 0.001$
Anhui	17.02	30.18	+13.16	$p < 0.001$
Xinjiang	15.60	29.20	+13.60	$p < 0.001$
Overall	18.54	31.36	+12.82	$p < 0.001$

TABLE C-6.3 PROVINCIAL AND OVERALL PRE- AND POST-TEST ANALYSIS OF CHINESE NURSES' KNOWLEDGE AND UNDERSTANDING OF HIV/AIDS WORK ENVIRONMENT EXPOSURE AND SELF-PROTECTION, 2006 (N = 643).

| Province | Mean Score | | Score Gain | Statistically Significant p Value |
	Pre-Test	Post-Test		
Yunnan	3.78	10.33	+6.55	$p < 0.001$
Guangxi	4.31	8.84	+4.53	$p < 0.001$
Anhui	4.56	8.41	+3.85	$p < 0.001$
Xinjiang	3.62	9.04	+5.42	$p < 0.001$
Overall	4.14	8.88	+4.74	$p < 0.001$

Although all three outcomes showed significant improvements, the differences in the score gains between provinces need to be explained to improve the effectiveness of the program. Whether the score gain differences result from differences in the participants' characteristics or contextual differences between provinces are questions that merit further analysis. Additional research and analysis will more clearly explain the differential performance.

UNEXPECTED CHALLENGES AND OPPORTUNITIES

A sustainable and growing network of Chinese nursing leaders has opened the door to increased communication and the establishment of new relationships that will potentially lead to resource sharing and collaborative research. This network evolved as nursing faculty from Xian Jiaotong and Sichuan Universities were prepared as trainers in 2004. Subsequently, nursing faculty from Sichuan University provided leadership in organizing the trainings in Yunnan and Guangxi provinces. Similarly, nursing faculty from Xian Jiaotong University organized the workshops in Anhui and Xinjiang provinces. Each of the faculties worked closely with the provincial nursing associations in selecting the nurses and coordinating arrangements for the venue and speakers. Nursing faculty also participated in workshop presentations and translated lectures given by international staff. Active participation in workshop activities provided an invaluable opportunity to "work across provinces" and network.

Some of the challenges and possible solutions include basic yet influential logistical concerns such as budgets, the number of participants in each group, dialect differences among participants, availability of local interpreters, translation of educational materials, and the selection of appropriate training facilities. Challenges are inevitable, and in China they have provided opportunities to improve and streamline subsequent training sessions.

Areas slated for further development as time and resources permit include the development of centers for excellence and academic nursing curriculum. Consideration will also be given for courses in addiction prevention—especially in Yunnan and Xinjiang provinces where intravenous drug use is a major vector in HIV transmission. Likewise, training initiatives in community care and palliative care should be undertaken, and demonstration models of community-based nursing programs should be established.

LESSONS LEARNED

- Use participant experience: In groups where nurses are actively involved in HIV/AIDS care, classroom time should be devoted to case study presentations that prompt discussion of issues faced in the workplace. These sessions should be conducted by clinical nurse experts familiar with standards of practice in China.

- Involve health policy leaders as well as practitioners: Local health authorities should always be invited to participate in training seminars to provided trainees with an accurate assessment of national and provincial HIV/AIDS prevalence rates and available medical services including the status of ARV distribution.

- Distribute as many resources as possible: Copying lectures to CDs is an easy and affordable method of providing students with lecture materials. When possible, presentations given by international faculty should be translated to Mandarin in advance of workshops for inclusion on the CDs.

- Engage: Interactive teaching/learning experiences should regularly be incorporated into training workshops as a method of advancing learning and preparing students for teaching in their home institutions.

WORDS OF WISDOM

Global Health Leadership initiatives at the University of Illinois at Chicago are designed to facilitate international learning opportunities for faculty and students. Overall interest in collaboration and research continues to grow, and all initiatives aim to ensure that such programs are of the greatest possible benefit to participants and to the communities with which they interact. Participatory engagement with local communities, sustainability, cultural appropriateness, quality learning, and safety should be priorities for all international work. Lessons learned through the China Nurses' Leadership Initiative for HIV/AIDS Care and Prevention may be applicable to other international work. Selected examples from China that may be relevant in other contexts are as follows:

1. Provincial universities that have assisted in supporting this initiative through faculty preparation and participation should be given support in developing distance-learning courses for technical nursing schools in their provinces. This can be accomplished

through web-based applications and will assist in meeting the demand for training for nurses who do not have ready access to major urban centers or universities for continuing education.

2. A methodology for conducting a long-term evaluation of the effects of training should be developed. Nurses who have completed the training should be surveyed or brought together for focus groups to determine how they have used the knowledge gained from training and how this has affected their places of work and communities. This would also provide an opportunity to determine the content and focus of future trainings.

3. Demographic information collected at each of the workshops should be maintained in a database for use by provincial and central nursing organizations. This database should be used when planning for future workshops and in inviting nurses to continue education in HIV/AIDS and/or related topics. This will lead to developing a cadre of nurse-experts that can be mobilized as trainers at the national and provincial level.

4. Provincial nursing associations and universities should be encouraged to meet for review and revision of the HIV/AIDS curriculum to stay current with advances in care and treatment in China.

5. Support should be provided for nurses associated with universities and teaching hospitals in urban settings to provide training for nurses in community settings, especially in rural areas where the majority of HIV/AIDS patients reside. Similarly, trained nurses should be given the opportunity to provide training at the village level for traditional healthcare workers who interact consistently with affected populations and have not been the focus of training efforts.

6. The central and provincial Chinese Nursing Association (CAN) should be encouraged to make the HIV/AIDS curriculum available in appropriate dialects to nurses representing minority populations.

REFERENCES

Joint United Nations Programme on HIV/AIDs. (2006). Retrieved 3 October 2007 from http://www.unaids.org/en/Regions_Countries/Countries/china.asp.

Reuters AlertNet. (27 November 2006). The price of blood in China: HIV/AIDS. Retrieved September 26, 2007 from http://www.alertnet.org/thefacts/reliefresources/116463687235. htm.

Acknowledgement: Several UIC WHO Collaborating Center personnel assisted in the preparation of this report including Shirley Stephenson, who provided editorial assistance; Chang Gi Park and Pei Yun Tsai, who provided data analysis, and Todd Hissong, who provided manuscript review.

7

INTERNATIONAL NETWORKING:
EXPANDING ONE'S WORLDVIEW

LARRY PURNELL, PhD, RN, FAAN

My penchant for travel and foreign places laid the groundwork for the creation of the Purnell Model for Cultural Competence, which was formalized in 1998. Little did I know at that time that a textbook on culture would exponentially increase my worldview through networking with people from throughout the United States and countries in Asia, Australia, Central and South America, and Europe.

As a poor, skinny, stubborn, sarcastic Appalachian child who had difficulty constructively directing his anger and impulses, I never expected to have the opportunity to become educated and achieve even a modicum of travel experiences, especially with scholarly endeavors, networking, presentations, and consultations. Although I made excellent grades in elementary and high school, to go beyond a bachelor's degree was not a consideration early in my career.

When I "escaped my roots" and started college, I gravitated to students from ethnicities, races, religions, and countries different from my own. I was fascinated by their descriptions of different places, different wildlife and plants, and foreign lands. When on school break from college, I always accepted invitations from other students to visit their homes. On one occasion, three of us drove to Acapulco, Mexico, to practice our Spanish, which at that time was my major. Thus, my interest in languages, travel, and different cultures was established.

During my second year in college, I redirected my educational efforts toward premed. However, a serious auto accident forced me to give up college for a semester. The patient experience intrigued me, and when I returned to school, I chose nursing. At that time, it was difficult to find a school that accepted men. Thus, I got an associate degree in nursing from Cuyahoga Community College in Cleveland, Ohio and then a bachelor's degree in nursing from Kent State University in Kent, Ohio. While speaking at the Michigan Male Nurses Association (MMNA), I met Luther Christman, an esteemed male nurse; he encouraged me to apply to Rush University in Chicago. After working in critical care and quality assurance for a few years at Rush Presbyterian St. Luke's Medical Center, I gravitated to administration, first in Chicago. Then, interestingly, I returned to Appalachia as the Chief Nursing Officer (CNO) at O'Bleness Memorial Hospital in Athens, Ohio. Twenty-five years later, Richard Castrop, the Chief Executive Officer of O'Bleness wrote, "I call Larry Purnell mercurial because he was a critical-care type guy and quite a character. He was a change agent. He pushed some of the nurses out of their comfort zones. Most responded—a few did not like it—and then he moved on" (Castrop, 2006).

I also started my doctorate in health services administration (PhD) via "distance initiatives" at Columbia Pacific University. At that time computers were not available for e-learning, and all assignments were through postal and telephone correspondence. With a PhD to my credit, I accepted a position in Washington, DC, as clinical director of critical care and shock trauma services. From there, I decided to teach, and for the last 19 years I have been at the University of Delaware where I direct the master of science (MS) and master of science in nursing (MSN) programs in health services administration and teach culture in the undergraduate and graduate programs in nursing as well as other departments.

RUNNING AWAY? OR RUNNING TO?

In my early childhood, I was accused of "running away" for days at a time in nearby forests. However, from my perspective, I was not running away, but rather, "running to" and exploring the country and watching wildlife. My first real trip out of Appalachia was a 4-day solo canoe trip through the Florida Everglades. I was a risk taker, not afraid of getting lost, and had a healthy respect for the wildlife and the people living in the Everglades. The next trip was the one to Acapulco to see indigenous tribes and, of course, Acapulco and Mexico City. Selected other travels beyond my academic career took me canoeing in the Amazon headwaters to see the Cofan Indians, to the Galapagos Islands, and on a 21-day trip through Europe where I saw 14 different countries (only the young can maintain this type of schedule). At the time, I had no idea that my travels would expand my worldview and prepare me for my eventual cultural diversity career.

OUTCOMES ACHIEVED

Teaching in a community hospital with patients and staff of Appalachian descent, I realized the need to include culture in the nursing curriculum. Because of the dichotomous relationship between students and staff, I started a framework for students to assess cultural attributes of their Appalachian patients. When staff saw the organizing framework, they became interested in it as well, so students and staff had joint post-clinical conferences on culture for the rest of the semester.

After a year of using the organizing framework, I recognized the need to further develop it. I also saw the need for staff to have comprehensive content covering all stages of life for specific cultures. For example, the migrant Mexican and Haitian populations working in farming, fishing, and the poultry industry became a challenge to staff. Information on health beliefs was readily available; however, little was found on death rituals and childbearing practices. Thus, I wrote a book describing an assessment model for cultural competence with cultural characteristics for ethnocultural specific groups. Although the original target audience was practicing staff, educators, administrators, and researchers began using the book as well.

PERSONAL SUCCESS MARKERS

My personal success markers include four networking accomplishments that have enriched my life. The first success marker was the opportunity to be a consultant in internationalization and cultural competence for the Benchmarking Internationalisation at Home in Undergraduate Nursing Education in Europe (BIHUNE) project of the European Union Commission's project of the Bologna–Sorbonne–Salamanca–WHO Declarations. The opportunity to work with faculty from 14 European countries was phenomenal. The second success marker was giving the keynote address at the 2nd International, 10th National Nursing Congress sponsored by Ege University in Izmir, Turkey. The third success marker was an invitation to give a keynote address, "Conceptual Concepts in Transcultural Health Care," at an International Multidisciplinary Transcultural Research Conference in Bogotá, Colombia, and to work with faculty and doctoral students who were completing their dissertations in culture. At the end of this week-long experience, I was named *padrino* (godfather) for the Transcultural Research Center (TRC) established at Universidad Nacional in Bogotá, Colombia. The fourth success marker was having my name carved on the Rosa Parks Wall of Teaching Tolerance in Montgomery, Alabama. These success markers are highlights of my personal experiences and professional career.

UNEXPECTED CHALLENGES AND OPPORTUNITIES

When I first started working with culture, I was unaware of the Transcultural Nursing Society (TNS). However, as I started reading about culture, an entire new world opened up to me which presented the opportunity to network with some wonderful people whose careers in culture preceded mine by decades; these individuals have been role models for many of us involved in transcultural nursing.

Perhaps the biggest challenge was developing the Purnell Model for Cultural Competence (PMCC) and making it comprehensive, non-prescriptive, and applicable to all health disciplines because much of the knowledge and skills required for cultural competence are needed by all healthcare providers. Within 2 years, the PMCC was an integral part of bachelor's, master's, and doctoral programs in nursing as well as in several medical schools and physical therapy programs. It was apparent that the PMCC required translation, first in French and then Spanish. Flemish, Portuguese, Turkish, and Korean versions soon followed. The model's acceptance enhanced my ability to network with other professional organizations and people from around the world, including Australia, China, Colombia, Costa Rica, Denmark, England, Finland, Hungary, Korea, Norway, Panama, Portugal, Russia, Scotland, Sweden, Turkey, and many schools of nursing in the United States (US).

LESSONS LEARNED

Even though theories and models are complex, they can be developed in such a way that, regardless of the educational level of the staff and students, they have value and components may be readily used by a diverse nursing audience. I have learned three very important lessons working with culture.

1. Give health professionals what they need, and they will use it and take it to dimensions beyond what you expected. For example, the staff wanted ethnocultural specific information, and they got it.

2. First, create something that is good for the patient; second, make it good for the nurse; third, make it good for the nursing profession; fourth, make it good for other professions; and fifth, make it good for the healthcare system. Everyone wins with culture.

3. Other countries are comparable within the area of culture. Their beliefs and practices are just as good, and sometimes better, than those from your own country. For some, their lack of resources does not allow them the luxury of disseminating their work through refereed journals and conferences like the US and some other countries.

WORDS OF WISDOM

Professional organizations and their members provide a wealth of information and are great networking resources. Become actively involved in at least two professional organizations. One should be broad in scope and cover all areas of nursing such as the American Nurses Association (ANA) and Sigma Theta Tau International (STTI). The second should be a specialty practice society such as the American Association of Critical-Care Nurses (AACN), American Organization of Nurse Executives (AONE), or TNS. Make sure at least one of the organizations has an international focus that facilitates crossing borders and networking with people globally.

You must move beyond your own comfort zone. Never approach another school or country with an ethnocentric attitude. Share what you know with them, but in a non-ethnocentric manner. Remember that learning transcends borders, and that everyone is both student and teacher. Thus, be open to critique of your work and add ideas you gain from their perspectives. When giving presentations or consulting in other schools and countries, remember their collective knowledge and wisdom is greater than yours. Take advantage of their knowledge and wisdom and share it with others.

CONCLUSION

Several years ago I asked colleagues, former students, and friends to describe me for a publication. Most of those asked were complimentary; however, the description that stood out was from my best friend, a retired federal judge. According to him, my mantra should be, "Why delay until tomorrow what I could have done yesterday." It is clear that he recognized my proactive approach to life and to life's experiences. My nursing career demonstrates that approach.

REFERENCE

Castrop, R. (2006). Managing O'Bleness Memorial Hospital. In G. Cordingley (Ed.), *History of medicine in Athens County Ohio* (231–250). Baltimore, MD: Gateway Press, Inc.

8

WRITING COLLABORATIVE

DIANNE RICHMOND, RN, MSN

MARIA HELENA LARCHER CALIRI, RN, PhD

LYN MIDDLETON, RN, PhD

"Whether you think you can or think you can't, you are usually right."
—Henry Ford

When nurses get together, great things are destined to happen. Such was the case in November 2005, during the Sigma Theta Tau International (STTI) Convention held in Indianapolis, Indiana, USA. A small group of nurses representing chapters from three different continents met casually for dinner. The attendees included Maria Helena Caliri (Brazil), Rosalina Rodrigues (Brazil), Leana Uys (South Africa), and Lynda Harrison and Pam Autrey of the United States (US). During the course of the evening Maria Helena Caliri mentioned the Brazilian faculty's desire to publish in peer-reviewed English language nursing journals. The primary language in Brazil is Portuguese. This alone was considered the most significant barrier to getting published in English nursing journals. Thus, the brainstorming began. It did not take long for this group to birth the idea of creating a virtual international writing collaborative with a mentoring focus. Two writing teams would be formed. Each team would consist of two members from each chapter, for a total of six members on each team. The goal of the writing collaborative would be to assist the 12 members in the production of a manuscript worthy of submission for publication. The collaborative would require a one-year commitment from all involved participants.

When the nurses returned to their respective chapters, the idea was received with great enthusiasm and anticipation by each chapter's board of directors and the deans of their respective schools of nursing. Each chapter identified a member to coordinate the activity of the writing collaborative. The selected coordinators were Maria Helena Caliri (Rho Upsilon Chapter, University of Sao Paula, at Ribeirao Preto, Brazil), Lyn Middleton (Tau-Lambda Chapter, University of KwaZulu-Natal, South Africa), and Dianne Richmond (Nu Chapter, University of Alabama at Birmingham, US.) The call to participate went out to both novice and experienced writers within each of the chapters. The member response to the call to participate was small but successful in all countries.

CREATING STRUCTURE

"The greatest problem in communication is the illusion that it has been accomplished."

—Daniel W. Davenport

The work of the coordinators unexpectedly extended the time it would take to actually implement the project. The combined visionary nature of the coordinators led them to seize the opportunity to create a blueprint for future replication by them and/or others. For the first 60 days e-mail exchange served as the mode of communication. Assignments were made; draft documents were created, circulated, and reviewed by each coordinator. Due to the inherent complexities of communication, the coordinators were careful to develop guidelines that would create a "meeting of meaning" that transcends cultural and language barriers. This effort resulted in the production of the Orientation Documents. The documents prepared for the Writing International Group (WIG) participants may be found in Table C-8.1.

TABLE C-8.1. COLLABORATION WRITING

Documents Prepared for the Writing International Group (WIG)
Welcome Letter
WIG Participant Responsibilities
Team Leader Responsibilities
Coordinator Responsibilities
Writing Assistive Mentor Responsibilities
Chat Room Access and Use
List of known Nursing Journals
WIG Etiquette
WIG Biographies
Copy of "Uniform Requirements for Manuscripts Submitted to Biomedical Journals"
Permission to Use Archives for Research Purposes
Consent to Use Archives for Research Purposes

During the process of creating the orientation documents an ambitious idea evolved. A suggestion was made to do a retrospective descriptive analysis of the project and submit it for publication. This required writing a research proposal and submitting it to the Institutional Review Board (IRB) equivalent in each country. It took 7 months to complete the IRB approval process required by each university. The pain of labor intensity was offset by the joy and excitement of task completion!

VIRTUALLY THERE

"It's kind of fun to do the impossible."
—Walt Disney

One of the most revolutionizing moments during the project planning phase was the moment that Dr. Lynda Harrison offered the use of the University of Alabama at Birmingham School of Nursing's Wimba chat room to the writing collaborative. Wimba provides an interactive virtual learning environment including a suite of online communications tools, called voice tools, voice discussion boards, and voice direct. All virtual interactions may be archived for future reference. Users may choose to interact using voice conferencing or text. The coordinators decided to use the text option for a number of reasons. 1) The text-based real time multi-user function created a sense of being present comparable to the voice option. 2) Though the Brazilians are proficient in reading and writing English, use of the spoken language presented a greater challenge because of the group composition of some participants who speak American English and some participants who speak British English. 3) Retrospective analysis of text data would be less time consuming than the analysis of voice data.

Three chat rooms have been established (one for each collaborative group and one for the coordinators). Archives of these meetings are stored on the School of Nursing Wimba site. Participants who are unable to attend any scheduled meeting are expected to review the archived meeting. The archived sessions will be used by the coordinators to complete the descriptive analysis of the overall process.

IMPLEMENTATION

"Man doesn't know what he is capable of until he is asked."
—Kofi Annan

Initially, a total of 13 nurses from the three chapters applied and were accepted for participation in the International Virtual Writing Collaborative Project. Five of the nurses were from the African chapter of STTI, four were from the Brazilian chapter, and four were from the American chapter. Two "virtual" writing groups were formed, one consisting of seven nurses and the other consisting of six nurses. The 13 nurse participants were assigned randomly to one of two groups. Each participant committed to working with the collaborative for a one-year period to develop a publishable manuscript and to assisting other group members with developing their manuscripts. The three chapter coordinators assisted in facilitating the project and coordinating activities over the 12-month period. Each group identified one member to act as the team leader. Six nursing professors, four Americans and two Brazilians, volunteered as mentors to provide academic guidance to the participants.

Each group meets in the virtual chat room at least monthly to discuss issues relevant to the manuscript development. Members may elect to have additional virtual meetings as needed. Virtual meetings held in the chat rooms are archived. Additionally, each member is required to review the manuscripts written by other members of their group and provide timely feedback. At the end of the 12 months, the coordinators review the archived data of the discussion sessions. Analysis of the data is used to document the process of initiating and implementing an international writing collaborative including strengths, weakness, barriers, and lessons learned. These data may ultimately be used as a part of a published document, PowerPoint presentation, abstract, or poster board.

Participants were apprised of the research activities and proposed use of archived data when orientation documents were disseminated for participant review before the virtual orientation sessions. Participants were provided opportunity to discuss use of archived data during virtual orientation sessions conducted by each chapter.

As of May 2007, the project work represents 6 months of planning and 9 months of implementation. Timeline adjustments have been required, but small successes leading to the overall goal have continued to energize the collaborative. Some of those milestones and successes are as follows:

1. Local virtual group meetings held, August 2006

2. All international participant virtual meeting held, September 2006

3. Received Sigma Theta Tau International Regional Showcase Award, September 2006

4. Group meetings begun, October 2006

5. Online "Manuscript Development" Presentation, November 2006

6. First drafts and outlines shared, December 2006

7. Mentorships formed, April 2007

8. Members of Group A submitted a jointly written manuscript to an online nursing journal, April 2007

9. Group A notified of *Southern Online Journal of Nursing Research* (SOJNR) acceptance of Group A's manuscript, May 2007

10. Abstract submitted to Sigma Theta Tau International biennial convention accepted April 2007

11. Institutional Review Board approvals from all three countries completed, April 2007

Participant drafts are in varying stages of near readiness for submission. Two participants have stated their inability to complete their manuscripts because of current competing priorities and obligations. We remain confident that many of the developed draft manuscripts will be accepted by peer-reviewed journals.

CHALLENGES AND OPPORTUNITIES

"A pessimist sees the difficulty in every opportunity; an optimist sees the opportunity in every difficulty."

—Sir Winston Churchill

Variation in time zones presented one of the greatest challenges for all chapters. The intercontinental differences in time zones could span as much as 8 hours. A 7-hour difference exists between U.S. Central Standard Time (GMT -5) and the time in South Africa (GMT +2). A 2-hour difference exists between Brazil (GMT -3) and the US (GMT -5). Arranging meeting times was further challenged by the daylight savings time changes in Brazil and the US that occur each year in November and March, which increases the time zone difference with South Africa by an additional hour.

Another challenge was keeping all members engaged in the process along the timeline. This was particularly challenging for the members of Group A that had the only true novice. This was further complicated by the fact that the novice did not work in an academic setting. All other participants had some experience with authorship and were academically attached. Unaware to other participants, this resulted in the novice's experiencing some group alienation

Keeping people connected and committed across three African countries—South Africa, Botswana, and Swaziland—has proved to be an unmet challenge. Some participants report difficulty in accessing the Internet, while others have dropped quietly off into cyberspace. Getting re-connected and working with members from the different African countries in developing nursing scholarship is an opportunity waiting to be embraced.

All of the participants from Brazil are nursing faculty from the same institution. The nursing school is home to the first Sigma Theta Tau International chapter in Latin America and has an active WHO Collaborating Center for Nursing Research Development. The writing collaborative has provided an opportunity for the participants to interact with their peers from other countries and cultures. Through this forum they have come to understand that their perceived barriers to getting published are universally related to personal and situational factors that must be recognized as we develop strategies to overcome them. The participants recognize that sharing lessons learned from their involvement in the writing collaborative could be of benefit to peers, students, and professional nurses in Brazil, Latin America, and African countries that have Portuguese as their native language.

The opportunities are endless. It is quite evident that eternal friendships have been created. Members of both groups have expressed interest in joint authorship around common themes that impact nursing in each country. It will be difficult at best to quantify or measure in any way the latent potential of such long term collaborative relationships. The overall impact is yet to be determined. However, it can definitively be stated that this forum provides an opportunity for all to teach and all to learn.

LESSONS LEARNED

"Failure is the opportunity to begin again, more intelligently."
—Henry Ford

One lesson learned is that mentorships should be created as early as possible and the mentors should be kept informed regarding the overall progress of the collaborative. We had almost a one-year gap from the time that the mentors committed to participate and the time that the mentors were actually assigned a participant. The newsletters that are prepared for the chapter board of directors could serve to keep the mentors informed on an ongoing basis and avert assumptions of project abandonment. Another lesson learned is that it may be beneficial to separate novice writers from experienced writers so that the pace of progression within each group can be tailored to group's composition. On the other hand, progression is only one among many of the variables that might be used to evaluate success. The benefits of working collegially in an experience-diverse group need to be explored for the extent to which this diversity shapes and enriches the scholarship of novice and experienced writers alike.

WORDS OF WISDOM

"There's an important difference between giving up and letting go."
—Jessica Hatchigan

Communities, like all life, are never static. They are adaptive organisms that are in a perpetual state of becoming. When one is in the midst of creating such organisms, one often seeks to attain the maximum levels of control over the process. But sometimes it is more beneficial to allow room for natural group evolution and adaptation. It is in these moments that one can experience the difference between giving up and letting go.

PART V

PRACTICE
SUCCESS STORIES

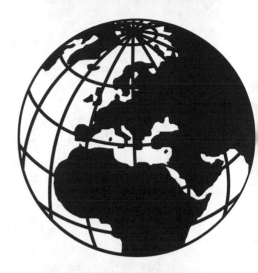

The practice of nursing spans generations as well as miles and mountains. Practice has changed dramatically since nursing's beginnings. These practice success stories are telling; they reveal dramatic and life-changing experiences that took the authors from the safety of their own environments to war zones and beyond. Their stories demonstrate advances in practice, enhanced outcomes, improvements in patient safety, standards, and certification. The global nursing leaders who have shared these remarkable stories have set the standard for each of us.

1

YEREVAN, ARMENIA: A STORY THAT MUST BE TOLD

MARIANNE E. HESS, BSN, RN, CCRN

On December 7, 1988, an earthquake struck Armenia, killing more than 25,000 people and injuring more than 16,000 people. Many countries and organizations came to the aid of Armenia including the Armenian General Benevolent Union (AGBU), which is a worldwide organization based in the United States (US). In 1989–1990, AGBU transported 62 earthquake patients to the US for specialized plastic and reconstructive surgery care, a discipline that was not fully developed in Armenia at that time. But, with so many earthquake patients, AGBU realized that they must instead bring this medical care to those in need. Therefore, AGBU arranged for a specially selected team of Armenian nurses, physicians, and biomedical personnel to come to Yale-New Haven Hospital, New Haven, Connecticut, for specialty education. Shortly after their return to Armenia, a U.S. health-care team joined them.

DESCRIPTION OF THE PROJECT

AGBU and the United States Agency for International Development (USAID) provided $2 million of funding for equipment and supplies to set up the Plastic and Reconstructive Surgery Center (PRSC) in Yerevan, Armenia. This state-of-the-art equipment would be used to establish two operating rooms (OR), a six-bed intensive care unit (ICU), and a 20-bed surgical floor in the Mikaelyan Surgical Institute. The PRSC's goals were to provide western treatment for such patients as those with post-earthquake wounds, congenital abnormalities, scar releases, and tendon and nerve grafts.

I was part of a four-person team from the US that included surgical nurse Carolyn Pritchyk, surgeon Dr. Paul Zamick, and project manager Mike McIntyre. We arrived in Yerevan in September 1992. Our mission was to establish a western-style center using train-the-trainer principles and to make the center self-sufficient.

OUTCOMES ACHIEVED

We performed our first surgical procedure in November 1992. To accomplish this we had to set up the OR, ICU, and surgical floor and organize the supply and medicine storage areas. In addition, we had to establish policies and standards of care for all three units. We developed medical record forms in Armenian and Russian. I educated the nursing staff on topics from electrocardiograms and malignant hyperthermia to vital signs and medication administration. Furthermore, we trained key personnel to train others, thus using the train-the-trainer principle. In addition to classroom-style teaching, we also taught by example. I precepted nurses in the ICU and surgical floor. We served as role models when performing nursing rounds, including displaying patient advocacy behaviors such as repeating patient privacy by knocking on doors before entering.

UNEXPECTED CHALLENGES AND OPPORTUNITIES

When I arrived in Armenia, it was one-year since Armenia declared its independence from the Soviet Union. Also, Armenia was at war with neighboring Azerbaijan, in the Nagorno-Karabakh region, and fuel and import embargoes were in place from other countries. This made living in Armenia challenging, and things were in a state of constant flux.

THE LOCAL SITUATION

Shortages of food produced bread lines; needed products or produce were not always available, nor affordable. Unemployment was overwhelming for many citizens. Intermittent supplies of water and electricity were a challenge. At my apartment, I never had hot water. In fact, I had only cold water and electricity on average of 4 hours a day, and I never knew when the 4 hours might occur. Sometimes I would have water, but no electricity or vice versa. Consequently, morning work conversation never addressed, "Did you watch that show on TV last night?" Instead, we would compare how much water or electricity we had. Utility outages certainly made life challenging, but constantly keeping the bathtub filled with water and using candles to read by helped. Armenia has four seasons, and the winters were difficult. There was never centralized heat in my apartment or in the hospital. In winter I could see my breath inside buildings. Some people could afford electrical or kerosene heaters, but many others were not as fortunate.

IMPACT ON THE HOSPITAL AND PATIENT CARE

The hospital also suffered from utility outages, although not as often or for as long. I carried a flashlight with me constantly and used it many times. With no hot water, surgeons scrubbed their hands with cold water.

Transportation was challenging. Public transportation was unreliable. Gasoline (benzene) was expensive and scarce. Many people walked to work or would crowd into over-stuffed vehicles. Yet, in spite of long, difficult commutes and utility outages, employees came to work. Their dedication always amazed me.

Communication was another obstacle. During electrical outages, phones didn't work, and the Internet was not yet established. So, we faxed most of our reports to AGBU. The language was a communication obstacle. Before arriving to Armenia, I did not speak any Armenian or Russian. The team that went to the US spoke fluent English. Staff tried to translate for me, but they were not always available. So, I decided to learn Russian because most of the medical chart and medications were in Russian. I got a good dictionary and used lots of non-verbal communication. A smile goes a long way in opening doors and creating relationships. I also used pictures to communicate. For example, rather than write the word "infant" in two or three languages, I cut out the picture of a baby from an empty box of Pampers® and taped it on the infant emergency box.

Nursing roles and responsibilities differ from that of the U.S. nurses. Because of differences in the Armenian nursing education, nurses in Armenia did not perform chest physical therapy, cardiopulmonary resuscitation (CPR), or a complete physical assessment—physicians did. Nurses were not responsible for feeding and bathing patients; family members assumed this role. Additionally, nurses stood up when physicians entered the room. Furthermore, many nurses and physicians worked 24-hour shifts; that was a difficult adjustment for me.

Supplies were another challenge for the project. Although ABGU worked hard at acquiring humanitarian aid, the goal was to make the unit self-sufficient. This meant we had to establish ways of getting supplies and medications in-country. We secured medications from Europe and former Soviet Republics. The medication names were unfamiliar to me and proposed a challenge. Also, because of availability and financial limitations, not every medication was accessible. The hospital even ran out of oxygen. The Armenians knew that these supply shortages were a hindrance, and they did all they could to prevent it.

Change can be a challenge, and Armenia was definitely going through a lot of it. For, a project to succeed there must be buy-in from everyone. Luckily, that was not a big obstacle for me because the PRSC staff was receptive to new ideas.

LESSONS LEARNED

Assess prior to diagnosing and implementing change. First, you have to make sure that this change will work in this culture. For example, I wanted the nurses to perform patient teaching, like nurses do in the US. But in Armenia, patients expect that the doctors will do that, not nurses. So, even though the nurses were ready for this change in practice, many of their patients were not.

Second, you have to make sure that the change will work in their infrastructure. For example, make sure that you buy electrical equipment with the right voltage (110 versus 220). Is there someone there who can routinely perform preventative maintenance on the equipment? Also, can you order more parts and supplies to fit that machine? With utility outages should your efforts be focused on a non-electrical solution until the country's infrastructure can support the use of electricity? Whether it is a new policy or piece of equipment, you have to make it work for you in your situation. Troubleshooting can be facilitated by contacting other organizations that are in-country to see how they are handling the infrastructure challenges. Why re-invent the wheel?

Third, remember the rationale behind why you do things a certain way. Is it research-based, or is it because you have always done it that way? For example, when transporting a patient on a gurney, is it feet first or head first? In the US I was taught "feet first" because the patients will get dizzy from not seeing where they are going. However, Armenians only transport patients "feet first" when they have died. So, I learned how to transport patients "head first." So, assess first, before diagnosing and changing something. Don't be judgmental. Reasons why things are done a certain way may exist. Instead, learn how to be more flexible and to "think outside of the box."

Follow the principles of adult learning. Teaching must be applicable to local learners. Teach them what they want to learn, and remember that issues in their personal lives like limited water and electricity, 24-hour shifts, and transportation problems, can make retaining this information more difficult. And in spite of my limited language abilities and lack of teaching materials (simulation labs, computers, LCDs), I was always amazed at the willingness of my colleagues to learn. To this day when I travel to Armenia to visit friends, they ask me when my next class will be. Furthermore, they loved *current* textbooks. If they have computers and electricity; however, I would take CD ROM textbooks instead, because textbooks can be very heavy. When taking teaching materials with you, keep it simple. You don't really need a Power-Point presentation to teach. I became very adept at drawing and teaching with my hands. My last CPR class was on a stuffed teddy bear. Granted, this is not ideal, but it worked.

Focus on the mission and don't get worn down by the challenges. Many of the impediments could not have been anticipated. Celebrate the large and small successes.

Advice to Others Considering International Work

My greatest advice is to accept the challenge. However, some things made my international work easier for me.

1. I had the support of my family, friends, and employer. (I cannot thank them all enough for this.)

2. I was prepared for the conditions. I don't know what I would have done without my flashlight and sturdy sleeping bag. Make sure that you are physically ready to go. I went to a travel clinic and got the required vaccinations. I went for my routine check-ups including dental and vision. At that time, it was difficult to obtain some items in Armenia, so, I took my own set of medical supplies (Motrin®, adhesive strips, even tampons) with me. I even made a will.

3. I kept a journal. Even when you are dead tired, write in your journal every day. I used it to document the events of the day, to log my expenses (especially helpful in an economy that was ever fluctuating), and to document photos I had taken.

4. I took a few items that reminded me of home. I took a few small Christmas decorations with me. That may sound unusual, but doing so helped bring the spirit of the holidays, even with just one decoration displayed. Also, I took a radio with me that could receive "Voice of America" and the "BBC" broadcasts. Before my departure to Armenia, I hesitated to buy the radio, thinking that it was a waste of money. My dad convinced me that I should get it. I never regretted taking his advice.

5. Assess before diagnosing and implementing a plan. Sound familiar? It's amazing how many times this plan is compromised.

I found my original notes to my director of nursing in Washington, DC, before my work in Armenia in which I asked, "Will you be upset if I come back early?" Needless to say, I had no idea this adventure would last longer than my initial six-month agreement. Amazingly, it extended into three six-month tours, on two surgical missions with Operation Smile, and included many trips back on my own to Armenia. The feeling of helping someone who is truly in need is incomparable. Whether you volunteer nationally or internationally, I encourage you to do something. The rewards outnumber the obstacles. Whether it is when a patient's mother kisses you on the cheek because you gave her child acetaminophen for a fever or when you see the joy on the face of a nurse who listened to the heart with a stethoscope for the first time, the feeling of really making a difference is exceptional. I hope that I will be able to do this again.

2

LITTLE THINGS REALLY DO MATTER: NEONATAL INTENSIVE CARE

CHRISTINE O. NEWMAN, MS, RNC, CNNP

With the fall of the iron curtain in the early 1990s, doors were opened for humanitarian missions in the former Soviet Union. The American International Health Alliance (AIHA), a consortium of major health-care provider associations and professional medical education organizations, was formed to help the nations of the former Soviet Union structure a much-needed health-care system. Funded initially by the United States Agency for International Development (USAID) through a series of cooperative agreements, partnerships linking U.S. hospitals with their counterparts in Georgia, Kyrgyzstan, Russia, Ukraine, and Uzbekistan were formed. Hospitals and organizations in the United States donated time and expertise of staff, and AIHA funded travel and expenses.

PARTNERSHIP PROCESS

The initial objective of these partnerships was to improve health care through education. The Henry Ford Health System (HFHS), Detroit, Michigan, was approached as one of the U.S. hospital systems to partner with the L'viv Oblast Clinical Hospital (LOCH) in western Ukraine. Several clinical partnerships resulted, one being the connection of Henry Ford Hospital's Newborn Intensive Care Unit (NICU) with the LOCH Premature Baby Unit.

After the facilities and clinical activities in L'viv were assessed by a neonatologist from HFHS, a neonatologist from LOCH came to Detroit for a 2-month training period. At the end of this period she identified not only clinical improvements in neonatal care that were necessary in the L'viv unit, but also the need to change the role of the bedside caregivers. At this time the medical director and the clinical nurse specialist from HFHS agreed to embark on what became a decade of opportunities to improve care to tiny infants in western Ukraine.

ASSESSMENT

An in-depth assessment made onsite in L'viv revealed that infants who survived in the district maternity hospitals were brought to this unit in L'viv for care that was impossible for them to receive in their birthplace. The facility at LOCH was a large 48-bed unit, which in 1993 had little capacity to provide much more than basic care to infants, and the mortality was high. Morbidities at this time were not quantified, but case reports depicted significant issues resulting from asphyxia, hypothermia, and other neonatal complications.

SUPPORT

Extensive support was needed to bring the facility at LOCH to our clinical standards. The partnership team collaborated to develop strategies and identify sources of support from within the Detroit and surrounding communities, along with a grant. AIHA and USAID provided support for basic educational exchanges. Special projects were also funded through small grants from USAID and HFHS. The need for outreach was clear, and partners reached out to the local Ukrainian community in the Detroit area and corporations for funding of equipment and supplies. One of the most significant partnerships developed was with a local Ukrainian organization in Warren, Michigan. The Ukrainian Village Corporation (UVC), a group of senior citizen Ukrainians, held annual benefits to support our efforts and to help give back to the country they loved so much. The people in the UVC literally adopted the tiny infants of western Ukraine and took pride in the lives they helped save.

Multitudes of professionals supported our Ukrainian colleagues on their clinical visits to Detroit. Their willingness to share knowledge and skills was overwhelming. Members of the Ukrainian community provided the much needed social support to the visiting nurses and physicians by arranging dinners and cultural activities to make them feel welcome and allowing them to experience life in the US. This contribution of human resources cannot be minimized in a partnership.

MAJOR ACHIEVEMENTS AND OUTCOMES

A three-tiered approach to improve care of infants in the region was developed: improve the clinical care of infants at the regional hospital by developing the capacity for providing intensive care; develop a transport system to safely move infants from the region to this unit earlier in their life; and develop a program for neonatal resuscitation and stabilization, to be used throughout the region so that during the first hours of life maximal support would be provided and neonatal outcomes would improve.

The unit in L'viv had been recognized as a referral center for many years, so the foundation for the partnership improvements was built on the concept of regionalization. We divided our efforts into four areas; clinical service, education, quality monitoring, and unit management. The components of each are depicted in Table P-2.1. Our initial efforts focused on the care provided in the unit.

TABLE P-2.1.   LEVEL III REGIONAL REFERRAL CENTER UNIT FOR PREMATURE AND SICK NEWBORNS.

Clinical Service	Quality Improvement
Clinical Care—infant and family	Data Collection and Evaluation
Support Services	Center Data
Transport Program	City Maternity Hospital Data
Follow-up Clinic	Regional Data
	Unit Quality Monitoring
Education	Unit Management
Neonatal Resuscitation Program	Roles and Responsibilities
Education for LOCH Staff	Committee Structure
Annual Conferences	
Outreach Education	
Family Education	

COLLABORATION

One of the significant differences identified between professionals at LOCH and in our U.S. unit was the remarkable separation of nurses and physicians. As leaders in the unit in Detroit, we had worked since the early 1980s to create a collaborative practice environment that was the foundation of our care to sick newborns and their families.

NURSING COMMUNITY

When I first entered the unit in L'viv with my physician colleague, I was excited to meet the members of the local nursing staff. I anticipated learning from them, and I was shocked when the bedside nurses left the room unannounced. No practice standards had been established for nurses, and nursing care consisted of basic tasks: feeding, clothing, and simple monitoring of infants. Nurses had no part in creating the plan of care with their physician colleagues. The stethoscope, an essential tool in U.S. nursing, was only a physician tool. In fact, routine nursing care provided in U.S. intensive care units was performed by physicians at LOCH. It was clear that we needed to develop strategies to break down these silos and help our Ukrainian colleagues create a model of practice that would improve not only technical care of infants, but also the quality of care and patient outcomes.

COLLABORATIVE PRACTICE

We believed collaboration would be essential to the unit's success. An essential component of acceptance of the change process is to engage all participants; all caregivers must understand and participate actively in the change. An environment supportive of change and growth is best cultivated if all staff are equally involved and seen as integral partners in this process. The educational exchanges in the US turned out to be one of the most successful strategies in pulling these professionals together. Physicians and nurses in equal numbers traveled together on these exchange visits. Not only did they witness how nurses and physicians interacted at the bedside, but these visitors also relied on one another as colleagues in this foreign country. This formed a bond that we saw carried over to the LOCH unit. A collaborative practice committee was established to help determine new standards of care and problem-solve issues related to the changes introduced. Both physicians and nurses participated in this structure.

Our philosophy of education also contributed to the collaborative effort. Because our focus has always been on preparing educational sessions targeted to a physician and nursing audience, our efforts for our partners were no different. We insisted nurses should be invited to all of the educational opportunities: rounds, lectures, and clinical skills demonstrations. The roles of both the physician and nurse were clearly delineated in all sessions, enabling both parties to understand the individual and collective roles of their colleagues within the clinical setting. Because the education was combined, everyone had the same foundation as a reference for clinical changes.

ROLE OF THE NURSE

To assist in the role transformation of the nurse, we requested and were granted permission by the hospital administrator to develop an additional leadership role for a nurse at LOCH. This second "head nurse" assumed the responsibility for educating nurses, overseeing clinical changes, and establishing standards for intensive care nursing. In the absence of formal nursing structure in this hospital, the development of this role was a significant step forward for the nursing staff. Nurses now use intensive care monitors to assist in their evaluation of infants, provide care for infants on ventilators, including managing the airway and troubleshooting issues. Nurses perform bedside laboratory testing and participate in daily rounds. We developed a bedside documentation system, which allows nurses to communicate vital clinical information to physicians. The nurse-patient ratio was changed from 1:8 in intensive care to 1:3.

Ironically, as the role of the nurse expanded, the physician role changed as well. Physicians began to assume responsibility for managing patient care and participated in clinical data collection to document patient care outcomes.

EDUCATION

Education was the foundation of our efforts and a springboard to success. Although we began with our colleagues from the L'viv unit—offering formal lectures and daily patient care teaching rounds, working side by side both at LOCH and HFHS with a multidisciplinary team of professionals, and scheduling clinical skills demonstrations—it was clear that we would be involved in outreach. Thus, the initial educational efforts expanded into regional efforts in Ukraine with visits to district hospitals with our colleagues from LOCH. These visits paved the way for a regional consultant role for the physicians at LOCH and led to clinical internships in the unit at LOCH by the district hospital nurses and physicians. Annual clinically focused conferences sponsored by HFHS, AIHA, and LOCH brought nurses and physicians from district and city hospitals together to learn about important topics in the care of sick newborns. Prior to our partnership efforts, multidisciplinary clinical conferences were not held in western Ukraine. Additional support came in the form of a translation of *The Newborn Care Manual,* our clinical guidelines from HFH, into Ukrainian. The fifth and sixth editions have been disseminated throughout L'viv and western Ukraine to physicians and nurses to guide their care of newborns.

TECHNICAL ADVANCEMENT IN CARE

An eight-bed intensive care unit was established in the unit at LOCH. Extensive networking with colleagues in Detroit, equipment vendors, and the serendipitous renovation of the NICU at HFH allowed us to fully equip the small intensive care unit with modern technology. Introduction of technology was not without problems; use of mechanical ventilation drained a meager oxygen supply, and voltage differences made transformers necessary. It was amazing that none of these issues created a major setback for our colleagues. Under the leadership of the unit director, they tackled problem after problem, advocating for what they needed to care for these infants. Today, the unit has been renovated, and adequate electrical supply supports the intensive care technology. Some of the advancements in place today are mechanical ventilation, regulated oxygen delivery, cardiorespiratory and oxygen saturation monitoring, controlled infusion therapy, and appropriate dosing and administration of medications. With the introduction of support services, blood gas machines, and electrolyte machines, care became data driven, which was important to improving the quality. As soon as the technological advances began to take hold, we concentrated on bringing infants to the unit safely and earlier in their lives.

TRANSPORT OF SICK NEWBORNS

A major focus of outreach education was the early transfer of sick infants from the region in an effort to decrease mortality and morbidity. Before our efforts, most infants arrived after 7 days of life, very sick and in almost every case hypothermic. Some who were kept warm with hot water bottles arrived severely burned. Transport was done by car when gasoline and a physician were available, and only if the infant survived the first few days. Ford Motor Company International (FMCI) donated a transit vehicle, and the UVC seniors raised money for an infant transport incubator. These two significant donations allowed us to put a program in place. The staff from LOCH could now go into the region and transport sick infants safely. Infants now mostly arrive on the first day of life, cared for during transport by trained intensive care staff.

NEONATAL RESUSCITATION

The resuscitation and stabilization of infants is tantamount to the transition to extra-uterine life and impacts long-term mortality and morbidity. Before our partnership, a German humanitarian group, Maltesier, worked with a Canadian nurse to begin the establishment of this program in L'viv. I was familiar with her efforts and contacted her. We built upon her initial efforts and established the first neonatal resuscitation training center in Ukraine at LOCH. Our colleagues, both physicians and nurses, were trained as instructors, and courses were offered monthly to caregivers in the city and region. In addition, donations of basic resuscitation equipment have been distributed to district hospitals to help the physicians and nurses implement these basic principles.

FOCUS ON PARENTS

For years, allowing parents to be involved in the care of their sick infant has been a struggle because of infection control beliefs. In the US, in the early years of neonatal care (1940s) parents could view infants only through a window. Over time, parents gradually entered the world of intensive care clothed in protective gowns and masks to prevent the spread of germs, and eventually, they were granted unlimited access to participate in their infant's care. At LOCH, mothers were housed in the hospital building but were not allowed in the unit to see their infants. They stayed to provide hand-expressed breast milk to feed the infants. Early on in the relationship, we introduced the concept of parent involvement as an important concept in the integration of a high-risk infant into the family structure. Though it took some time, mothers now nurse or feed their infants milk from a bottle in the unit and interact daily with their infants, and nurses teach the new moms how to care for them.

EVALUATION OF PROGRAM OUTCOMES

A computer database program was developed to allow for query of clinical outcomes of care. Clinical information extracted from patient charts was entered by physicians at the time of discharge of an infant. This data was used to trend newly instituted clinical practice changes and their impact on outcomes. Modifications in care could be made based on results. Internet and computer support established regular communication between the partners and kept our efforts alive even when we were not onsite in L'viv.

UNEXPECTED CHALLENGES

Although there were many challenges that our partners faced daily in their efforts to improve neonatal care, there were two significant ones. Local culture derived as a result of years under communist rule led to a generalized "acceptance" of events and circumstances. Our colleagues accepted obstacles, especially "official obstacles," and early on, when we questioned them, they would often say, "This is just the way it is." Although an item might be needed to improve clinical outcomes, challenging those in authority seemed inappropriate. Initially, we assumed the advocacy role, requesting support and items that were needed for the care of these babies. As our colleagues observed our problem-solving tactics and strategies, they assumed this advocacy role. Asking for what was needed for the vulnerable patients for whom one provided care enhanced our colleagues' self-esteem and courage. Our constant support added an ingredient that helped our counterparts develop into the best advocates for the unit.

The other cultural obstacle we encountered was our realization that public health rules and regulations govern care and are enforced as law. Deviations from these rules could lead to punishment of the person(s) involved. This often impeded changes in the unit, and we used much time to negotiate with officials just to make simple improvements. Partnerships are based on relationships; the relationship that we established with the administrative head of LOCH was tantamount to our success. She often intervened in eliminating obstacles to care delivery.

LESSONS LEARNED

In the US, as leaders of a NICU, we were constantly striving to improve care by adopting new strategies based on research and literature. Our assumption was that we would do the same in L'viv. It took time to understand that guidelines and standards of care in this country were established by the Ministry of Health (MOH), a local health administration, and accepted research did not always serve as a basis for practice standards. Proposed changes did not always coincide with the agenda of local officials, and we developed strategies to gain their support.

Education without resources was a source of frustration for our colleagues and was often a barrier to improving patient outcomes in the unit. Without material resources, little change can be made. Although our initial charge was to provide education, we quickly determined the need for equipment and supplies and became advocates and curators of items needed in L'viv. Millions of dollars of aid was collected and shipped over the 10 years of our partnership and continues to this day.

Communication is critical to the life and growth of a partnership. In the beginning, little access to the Internet was available, and the only means of communication was by phone. Our personal investment early on in a computer and Internet connection was one of the best strategies we employed. This means of communication between the partners gave us not only a constant connection for continued dialogues regarding issues, but also provided a connection for clinical consultation.

Commitment is essential and not without personal sacrifice. This partnership was a lifeline for our professional colleagues as well as the infants entrusted to their care. They often shared their concern that many people came to visit and promised to help, but few followed through. This made it clear to us that our commitment needed to be without wavering and was one of the most important things to enhance our colleagues' growth and independence. Our continued commitment eliminated their constant explaining of issues to every new group of people and created a seamless approach to the project.

WORDS OF WISDOM

- **Understanding of the local culture is critical to success.** This understanding often takes time. People rarely reveal all details, especially those problems that might be looked upon as unfavorable, until a trusting relationship is established. Most people want to improve their situation, but an outsider must understand the local climate, obstacles, and realities to help effectively. Basic concepts may be the same, but how you implement and make any change is different in different environments.

- **Develop a detailed plan** *with* **the partners**—do not develop a plan for them. They must be equal partners and understand and determine what is needed in their environment.

- **Consistency of a core group of people that are committed to the project is essential as it builds trust and prevents rework and allows you to focus on the plan developed.** If you make a commitment, make sure you *follow through*. Only then is there trust, and development of trust is essential to success.

- **Empower the people.** It is important to provide support to the people in their environment in which work and change is being made. With support most people will strive to improve, knowing that they can fall back on others if needed. Regardless of the side of the partnership you are on, you have a lot to learn from one and other. *Partners that grow together can establish long-lasting partnerships.*

Special thanks to my colleagues in L'viv Ukraine, Henry Ford Hospital Newborn Intensive Care Unit, and my mentor, Sudhakar Ezhuthachan, MD, for giving me this opportunity and allowing me such professional and personal growth.

3

MAGNET JOURNEY TO BRISBANE

JENNIFER ANDREWS, RN, ADON
JEANNE M. FLOYD, PhD, RN, CAE, FAAN

The Magnet Recognition Program® (MRP) represents a journey for those hospitals that seek this special designation. That journey has reached beyond United States (US) borders and is now an important part of nursing recognition in many countries, including one as diverse as Australia. We share our experience in seeking Magnet Recognition, and the impact that it has made on our facility. The MRP seeks to advance three goals within each applicant and designee:

- Promoting quality in a setting that supports professional practice

- Identifying excellence in the delivery of nursing services to patients/residents

- Disseminating "best practices" in nursing services

The MRP is a credentialing program developed by the American Nurses Credentialing Center (ANCC) to recognize health-care organizations that provide nursing excellence. This includes a broad spectrum of health-care facilities committed to improved nursing care by meeting research-based standards of care and professional performance. The original Magnet research study from 1983 first identified 14 characteristics that differentiated organizations that were best able to recruit and retain nurses during the nursing shortages of the 1970s and 1980s. These characteristics became the ANCC Forces of Magnetism that provide the conceptual framework for the Magnet appraisal process. See Table P-3.1.

TABLE P-3.1.   FORCES OF MAGNETISM

Described as the heart of the MRP, the Forces of Magnetism exemplify excellence in nursing. Designation as a Magnet facility requires compliance with the 14 Forces.

Force 1: Quality of Nursing Leadership

Knowledgeable, strong, risk-taking nurse leaders follow a well articulated, strategic, and visionary philosophy in the day to day operations of the nursing services. Nursing leaders, at all levels of the organization, convey a strong sense of advocacy and support for the staff and for the patient. *(The results of quality leadership are evident in nursing practice at the patient's side.)*

TABLE P-3.1.   FORCES OF MAGNETISM (CONTINUED)

Force 2: Organizational Structure

Organizational structures are generally flat, rather than tall, and decentralized decision making prevails. The organizational structure is dynamic and responsive to change. Strong nursing representation is evident in the organizational committee structure. Executive-level nursing leaders serve at the executive level of the organization. The Chief Nursing Officer typically reports directly to the Chief Executive Officer. The organization has a functioning and productive system of shared decision making.

Force 3: Management Style

Health-care organization and nursing leaders create an environment supporting participation. Feedback is encouraged and valued and is incorporated from the staff at all levels of the organization. Nurses serving in leadership positions are visible, accessible, and committed to communicating effectively with staff.

Force 4: Personnel Policies and Programs

Salaries and benefits are competitive. Creative and flexible staffing models that support a safe and healthy work environment are used. Personnel policies are created with direct care nurse involvement. Significant opportunities for professional growth exist in administrative and clinical tracks. Personnel policies and programs support professional nursing practice, work/life balance, and the delivery of quality care.

Force 5: Professional Models of Care

There are models of care that give nurses the responsibility and authority for the provision of direct patient care. Nurses are accountable for their own practice as well as the coordination of care. The models of care (i.e., primary nursing, case management, family-centered, district, and holistic) provide for the continuity of care across the continuum. The models take into consideration patients' unique needs and provide skilled nurses and adequate resources to accomplish desired outcomes.

Force 6: Quality of Care

Quality is the systematic driving force for nursing and the organization. Nurses serving in leadership positions are responsible for providing an environment that positively influences patient outcomes. There is a pervasive perception among nurses that they provide high-quality care to patients.

Force 7: Quality Improvement

The organization has structures and processes for the measurement of quality and programs for improving the quality of care and services within the organization.

Force 8: Consultation and Resources

The health-care organization provides adequate resources, support, and opportunities for the utilization of experts, particularly advanced practice nurses. In addition, the organization promotes involvement of nurses in professional organizations and among peers in the community.

Force 9: Autonomy

Autonomous nursing care is the ability of a nurse to assess and provide nursing actions as appropriate for patient care based on competence, professional expertise, and knowledge. The nurse is expected to practice autonomously, consistent with professional standards. Independent judgment is expected to be exercised within the context of interdisciplinary and multidisciplinary approaches to patient/resident/client care.

Force 10: Community and the Health Care Organization

Relationships are established within and among all types of health-care organizations and other community organizations, to develop strong partnerships that support improved client outcomes and the health of the communities they serve.

Force 11: Nurses as Teachers

Professional nurses are involved in educational activities within the organization and community. Students from a variety of academic programs are welcomed and supported in the organization; contractual arrangements are mutually beneficial. There is a development and mentoring program for staff preceptors for all levels of students (including students, new graduates, experienced nurses, etc.). Staff in all positions serve as faculty and preceptors for students from a variety of academic programs. There is a patient education program that meets the diverse needs of patients in all of the care settings of the organization.

Force 12: Image of Nursing

The services provided by nurses are characterized as essential by other members of the health-care team. Nurses are viewed as integral to the health-care organization's ability to provide patient care. Nursing effectively influences system-wide processes.

Force 13: Interdisciplinary Relationships

Collaborative working relationships within and among the disciplines are valued. Mutual respect is based on the premise that all members of the health-care team make essential and meaningful contributions in the achievement of clinical outcomes. Conflict management strategies are in place and are used effectively, when indicated.

Force 14: Professional Development

The health-care organization values and supports the personal and professional growth and development of staff. In addition to quality orientation and in-service education addressed earlier in Force 11, Nurses as Teachers, emphasis is placed on career development services. Programs that promote formal education, professional certification, and career development are evident. Competency-based clinical and leadership/management development is promoted and adequate human and fiscal resources for all professional development programs are provided.

Reprinted with permission from Margaret L. McClure and Ada Sue Hinshaw, editors, Magnet Hospitals Revisited: Attraction and Retention of Professional Nurses, © 2002 Nursesbooks.org, Silver Spring, MD.

PRINCESS ALEXANDRA HOSPITAL HEALTH SERVICE DISTRICT

The Princess Alexandra Hospital (PAH) is one of three tertiary level facilities in Queensland, providing care in all major adult specialties with the exception of obstetrics, and one of Australia's leading teaching and research hospital. In 2004, the staff of PAH were elated to be the first hospital in the Southern Hemisphere to receive the prestigious Magnet designation for excellence in nursing care.

PAH has 2,000 outstanding nursing staff who have undergone this rigorous, voluntary, in-depth evaluation process to examine nursing services, and we are proud of our recognition. On the local level, the MRP offered a framework through which the nursing environment and culture are analysed. It sets the benchmark for constantly reviewing and improving our practices to ultimately improve patient outcomes, which is always the hospital's goal.

In support of this process, PAH developed an electronic workbook that addresses each of the 14 Magnet Forces, which align with the Australian Council of Health Care Standards. This tool provides nurses with the autonomy to analyse, review, and instigate work place changes. Nurses have also implemented unit-specific scorecards focusing on patient outcomes. This provides evidenced-based data to support practice and allows nurses to analyse and benchmark indicators.

DESCRIPTION OF PROJECT

PAH representative, Jennifer Andrews, assistant director of nursing in the division of surgery, shared the Magnet journey of Princess Alexandra Hospital. Princess Alexandra Hospital is one of Australia's leading teaching hospitals, providing all adult specialties with the exception of obstetrics. With approximately 750 beds, it serves a large and diverse patient population, providing clinical, educational, and research leadership across the southern zone of the state of Queensland and northern New South Wales.

MAGNET JOURNEY AND OUTCOMES

The benefits that we have experienced include allowing our staff to reflect on their practice, giving them permission to be innovative and reflective of practice, and offering continual opportunities to reflect on and improve all aspects of practice. We invested time, resources, effort, and commitment to the ongoing evolution, and we know that the interim monitoring process ensures continuity. Our nurses share their thoughts:

> I have worked in ward 4A Urology at the [Princess Alexandra Hospital] PAH since completing my nursing training in 1991. I have seen enormous change within that time, both good and bad, as anyone would. Since commencing the Magnet journey in 2000, I have noted radical changes in the way nursing staff are actively and positively involved in processes that determine patient outcomes. I think that we really needed to do this [Magnet recognition] as a profession to bring us together as a cohesive group, a powerful group, a group of people aware of patient needs and able to effect change. Magnet has given us a sense of control, and we have autonomy in our profession today, even with the most junior staff member actively involved in change at ward level. I think working in a Magnet recognized hospital—indeed the only hospital in Australia with Magnet recognition—makes us proud, encourages us to do better, to excel.
>
> —CN Glen Waller, Ward 4A

> For the past six years, I have worked as a renal nurse at the Princess Alexandra Hospital. I have been a Magnet champion since the inception of our journey, and I admit it has been demanding, but it has been more rewarding than words can describe. It is inspiring to realise that you can effect change for your patients and staff within your ward and organisation from a clinical level. The [Magnet Recognition Program] MRP has given all of our nurses that opportunity.
>
> —CN Shannon Glass, Magnet Champion

UNEXPECTED CHALLENGES

As you can imagine, the challenges facing an international facility seeking Magnet status are real. First of all, the cost involved was significant; however, we chose to focus not on what it cost, but rather on what it saved in terms of outcomes and staff retention. Language barriers also presented a challenge. Terms such as *components/objectives, interdisciplinary/multidisciplinary, sources of evidence/goals*, and *staff scheduling/rostering* and acronyms such as *CNO/EDNS* are used interchangeably. With respect to data collection, PAH information systems were insufficient to meet the Magnet requirements and continue to pose a challenge.

The human resources and information systems departments, which are dictated by Australian requirements, also found the terminology to be used quite different. And, *benchmarking* at the national and international levels is not a familiar term.

LESSONS LEARNED

Despite presenting significant challenges for a non-U.S. facility, the journey to excellence had been very successful for us. Before we began the Magnet journey, we suffered critical nursing shortages. The change in the environment of the organization resulting from the Magnet experience has been a key factor in alleviating this situation and has brought many other benefits.

WORDS OF WISDOM TO OTHERS SEEKING INTERNATIONAL MAGNET RECOGNITION

Focused on nursing as an essential service, this journey is within the reach of acute and primary health-care facilities regardless of their geographic location and has been modified for universal application. The status is not permanent; facilities must be redesignated at predetermined intervals. But, the Magnet journey is well worth the outcomes!

REFERENCE

American Nurses Credentialing Center. (n.d.) *Forces of Magnetism*. Author. Retrieved 27 September 2007 from http://www.nursecredentialing.org/magnet/forces.html.

4

A CAPITAL TRANSFORMATION

TIM PORTER-O'GRADY, DM, EdD, APRN, FAAN

At the turn of the century the Capital and Coast District Health Board, Wellington, New Zealand (NZ), determined a major transformation of their health system was in order. New administration and clinical leadership including a new chief nurse executive (CNE) were hired to provide fresh new direction for the health system, including a brand-new patient care facility in the capital city of Wellington. The Wellington Hospital had come in existence early in the 20th century and had a long history of tradition and entrenchment in past practices across the medical and clinical services, including the nursing services. The board's major commitment to the Wellington Hospital transformation and the planning and construction of a new facility, along with new leadership, drove a breath of fresh air into the organization and acted as a harbinger of considerable change throughout the organization.

PLANNING FOR THE FUTURE

The CNE was determined to build a strong nursing strategy based on creating a contemporary 21st-century nursing organization with a professional frame and representing the foundation upon which more relevant practice concepts and processes could be constructed (Porter-O'Grady, 2001a). The CNE came to the United States (US) to expand the nursing organization's understanding of newer professional models, shared governance, and new foundations for excellence in clinical practice. She connected with Tim Porter-O'Grady Associates, Inc., and worked with Dr. Tim Porter-O'Grady to clarify the strategic and process foundations for transforming the nursing organization at the Capital Coast Wellington Hospital and preparing the nurses to move from the very old architectural infrastructure toward a completely redesigned patient care delivery model (Joel & Kelly, 2002).

While in the US, the CNE and her visiting team were scheduled to visit a number of different hospitals noted for their excellence in patient care, leadership, and shared governance as a vehicle for helping inform the leadership team from NZ with regard to the best organizational and nursing practices in the US. The same time as the hospital visits were conducted, strategic conversations and analysis was undertaken and applied to the unique characteristics of the Wellington Hospital. A major consideration was the reflection of cultural, conditional, and professional differences between nursing practices in NZ and those reviewed in the US (LeBaron, 2003). Included in those critical discussions were issues related to differences in nursing education, expectations for clinical practice, processes and content of nursing clinical activities, and interprofessional relationships; also, social, cultural, and gender differences between the two countries were detailed and clarified (Hultman & Gellermann, 2002). Additionally, the relationship between medicine and nursing in U.S. hospitals and NZ hospitals was contrasted as a part of determining the facilitators and constraints related to building a truly professional, equity-based nursing organization at the Wellington Hospital.

BUILDING STRONG STRATEGIC FOUNDATIONS

The conversations and strategic priorities established by the visiting Wellington Hospital nursing leadership team formed the foundations for subsequent leadership activity that would be initiated upon their return to the Wellington Hospital. It was also decided that Dr. Porter-O'Grady would make a consultation visit to Wellington Hospital to assist them in translating strategy, tactics, and methodology for application and change within the cultural context of Wellington Hospital (Pietersen, 2002). In addition, other consultants familiar with clinical systems change and the achievement of excellence exemplified by the Magnet Recognition Program would follow over time to help continue the development efforts for nursing at the Wellington Hospital. Critical elements of the planned activities and stages of implementation were as follows:

1. Reformat and restructure the nursing leadership team to position leaders able to undertake the challenges and vagaries of a major shift in the culture and condition of nursing practice at the hospital.

2. Decentralize the locus of control and units of service reflecting a stronger service line orientation yet strengthening nursing's decision-making capacity in partnership decisions affecting structure, process, and delivery of patient care.

3. Develop a strong first-line management team with the new leadership skills necessary to re-conceive, redefine, and apply new or contemporary approaches to patient care and clinical practice and to anticipate changing professional requirements in a new facility.

4. Introduce the concepts and begin the initial structure of shared governance and shared leadership development in the nursing service as a way of strengthening the point-of-service decision-making capacity of the professional nurse.

5. Strengthen and improve the nurse-physician relationship and evidence that relationship by forging a stronger formal infrastructure between medicine and nursing and increasing the intensity of the decision-making role of the nurse in a previously medically dominated decision-making environment.

6. More specifically address the historic, cultural, role, and behavioral characteristics of the profession of nursing with an aim at changing performance expectations, role definitions, job descriptions, and dress codes to represent a more contemporary nursing-driven clinical environment.

7. Build stronger more equity-based relationships at the administrative level between the CNE role and the other senior roles in the organization as a way of better positioning nursing in the organizational decision process and in creating an opportunity for stronger nursing influence in decision-making for the organization.

Upon appointment, that new senior nursing leadership team incorporated these strategic imperatives into their initial activities as they began the effort to transform the nursing organization in preparation for new practice models and a new clinical facility. The timetable and plan of activities representing the preceding factors were outlined by the senior nursing leadership team, providing a framework for subsequent actions, implementation, and evaluation of the significant cultural and practice changes in the organization (Mische, 2001). Considerable initial effort was focused on enhancing and advancing leadership team skills and providing a new foundation for leadership practice that would represent more shared leadership and shared governance practice behaviors across the profession and throughout the nursing organization (Porter-O'Grady, 2001b)

CONFRONTING HISTORY AND CULTURE

Early successes were difficult to obtain. Considerable historic entrenchment and a high volume of long-term employment served to create a strong level of organizational stasis (Light, 2005). Difficulties in the new leadership conception, translation, and application of changed leadership roles took much longer than initially expected. This condition was driven not so much by a lack of willingness, but more by a lack of understanding and application. Previous practice patterns and behavioral models were well established and strongly entrenched in the roles and behavioral patterns of the nurses, physicians, and other practitioners, as well as administrators. Challenges were met on all fronts, each requiring detailed conversation and process changes. Each of these also required continuous re-explanation and validation to eventually get buy-in and broader-based support. The organization was loathe to embrace experimentation, and the organization's historic lack of listening often acted as a major impediment to transitioning toward new practices.

At the other extreme, nursing staff began with strong initial successes in making decisions, changing practices, participating strongly in decision-making, and engaging and embracing new professional processes. Staff readiness for major change reflected a long pent-up history of disenfranchisement and lack of empowerment within the traditional organization (Huffington, 2004). Once freed of these constraints, the staff enthusiastically, even exuberantly, began to embrace their own developing and growing role as full active professionals. At the same time, these patterns of behaviors, while positive, created their own negative organizational reaction. Administrators and managers, unable to keep up with the leadership requisites of staff-driven decision-making, tended to constrain and limit the staff in terms of the range of permissible decision-making (Parker, 2003). Leadership's incapacity to cope with the growing professional self-direction and confidence created a potentially damaging damper on the energy and pace of staff professional development.

Leadership development and maturation was accelerated with a great deal of administrative and educational support as a way of enabling first-line leader's capacity to address the staff's growing decision-making competence. Also, strengthening the infrastructure of shared leadership and shared governance helped create a format and specific forums within which the components of decision-making and the specific accountabilities related to particular decisions could be better classified and categorized. Those decisions that were specifically and clearly management driven could then be separated from clinical and staff-driven accountabilities for decision-making and clarified in a way that would identify specific decision accountabilities and delineate the interfaces between varying categories of decision-making (Hickman, Smith, & Conners, 2004). Finding the intersections between council accountability, individual management performance expectations, and unit-driven decision-making helped more appropriately determine the parameters of decision-making and the points of facilitation necessary to assure successful application across the nursing organization.

Subsequent consultant visits from Dr. Porter-O'Grady and other consultants helped the nursing organization more specifically clarify its strategic priorities, tactical initiatives, and cultural challenges and delineate better mechanisms to address them. Continual exploration and dialogue between historic realities and transformational expectations helped both staff and leaders identify and anticipate challenges and difficulties in unfolding a more contemporary framework for decision-making and practice. Furthermore, specific issues with regard to medical staff integration and administrative support of nursing practice changes were also identified and incorporated into the planning and application activities of nursing senior leadership and the newly emerging nursing councils.

LESSONS AND NEW WISDOM

Initiating a significant cultural change and nursing organization in NZ is certainly not the same as initiating those same changes in hospitals in the US. An organization built in a country sharing a common history, language, and broad culture does not necessarily successfully translate into application in nations that are separated by the great distance of unique experiences, specific population characteristics, a defined social, political, and professional infrastructure, and a different medical infrastructure (Earley & Mosakowski, 2004). While it is clear that principles are consistent across populations and cultures, their application must reflect the unique characteristics of national and local realities that reflect a more specifically delineated professional journey. Many of the nursing values and insights with regard to professionalism and application are similar between the US and NZ. However, the rate of change, cultural expectations, gender issues, and medical models are different between the two nations and create an entirely different configuration representing the current conditions and progress in each nation.

Clearly, the most significant differences between implementing nursing professional change in the US and NZ in this case related to history, gender, and structure. It is important to those undertaking international work to recognize that these specific areas of difference will have a common frame of reference regardless of the nation an international consultant will be working within. The US represents a particular model of cultural and social change, reflecting its own history and developmental experiences. In NZ, cultural, social, political, and gender development have followed a uniquely different path, requiring understanding and modifications of those practices in applications taken to NZ from the US. Furthermore, NZ is a small nation of between 3 and 4 million people. It reflects greater sensitivity to any change implemented in one component of the health system and its potential implications for the entire health system. This is clearly not an issue in the US, a nation of more than 300 million people.

Much of the initial activity undertaken to professionalize the nursing staff at the Wellington Hospital and prepare them for a change to a new facility was exceptionally successful. However, many of the setbacks and challenges to the pace of change were driven as a direct result of the conflict between the differences in application between the social and professional culture of NZ's nursing when separated from that of American nursing. An earlier recognition of these realities and a quicker incorporation of the cultural vagaries and realities of the NZ nurse's experiences could have shortened and limited the intensity of reaction to many of the initial changes. However, when successfully translated and incorporated within the cultural, political, and social framework of NZ health care, the changing and maturing practices and self-direction of the nursing profession at Wellington Hospital was facilitated and positively encouraged.

REFERENCES

Earley, C. & Mosakowski, E. (2004). Cultural intelligence. *Harvard Business Review, 82*(10), 139–146.

Hickman, C., Smith, T., & Conners, R. (2004). *The Oz Principle: Getting results through individual and organizational accountability*. New York: Portfolio Hardcover.

Huffington, C. (2004). *Working below the surface : the emotional life of contemporary organizations*. London, New York: Karnac.

Hultman, K. & Gellermann, W. (2002). *Balancing individual and organizational values : walking the tightrope to success*. San Francisco: Jossey-Bass/Pfeiffer.

Joel, L. A. & Kelly, L. Y. (2002). *The nursing experience : trends, challenges, and transitions* (4th ed.). New York: McGraw-Hill.

LeBaron, M. (2003). *Bridging cultural conflicts : a new approach for a changing world* (1st ed.). San Francisco: Jossey-Bass.

Light, P. C. (2005). *The four pillars of high performance : How robust organizations achieve extraordinary results*. New York: McGraw-Hill.

Mische, M. (2001). *Strategic renewal : Becoming a high-performance organization*. Upper Saddle River, NJ: Prentice Hall.

Parker, G. M. (2003). *Cross-functional teams : working with allies, enemies, and other strangers* (2nd ed.). San Francisco, CA: Jossey-Bass.

Pietersen, W. (2002). *Reinventing strategy*. New York: Wiley Publishers.

Porter-O'Grady, T. (2001a). 21st Century strategic thinking: Five Insights for Boards of Trustees. *Health Progress,* 28–46.

Porter-O'Grady, T. (2001b). Is Shared Governance Still Relevant. *Journal of Nursing Administration, 31*(10), 468–473.

5

A PORTUGUESE EXPERIENCE WITH ICNP®

ABEL PAIVA, MSN, PhD, RN
AMY COENEN, PhD, RN, FAAN
CLAUDIA BARTZ, PhD, RN, FAAN

The International Classification for Nursing Practice (ICNP®) is a program of the International Council of Nurses (ICN). ICN's mandate is to improve the health of the world's people by improving nursing practice, education, management, and research and strengthening nurses' contribution to health systems at all levels. ICNP is a tool to assist collection and comparison of data across clinical settings, client populations, geographic areas, and languages. Development of ICNP began in 1989 and Version 1.0 was launched at the 2005 ICN Congress in Taiwan. The ICNP vision is to be an integral part of the global information infrastructure, informing health-care practice and policy to improve patient care worldwide. Major structural changes were made with Version 1.0 with the aim of making it a universal nursing language that could promote a shared meaning of concepts in nursing, thus facilitating documentation of comparable data for use in health information systems and electronic health records (EHRs).

The need and desire for a standardized language for medical records is nothing new. Florence Nightingale began the movement in this direction. Recognizing the need for defining nursing's role, contributions, and unique body of knowledge eventually led to the development of a classification of nursing diagnoses.

In 1973, Kristine Gebbie and Mary Ann Lavin called for the first task force to name and classify nursing diagnoses. The Task Force of the National Conference Group on the Classification of Nursing Diagnoses was formed in 1974. In 1982, the North American Nursing Diagnosis Association (NANDA) was created, incorporating National Task Force members from the United States (US) and Canada. By 1986, NANDA created a classification system that labeled and articulated nursing diagnoses (North American Nursing Diagnosis Association, n.d.).

Although the acronym NANDA stands for the organization, it is commonly used to refer to the language itself and will be used here to denote the language. The concept of nursing diagnosis is a successful clinical initiative, and nursing diagnosis is internationally accepted as a critical step in a systematic and individualized care plan.

NANDA nomenclature represents clinical nursing judgments about actual or potential health problems. NANDA diagnoses describe a patient's reaction to disease or injury and could be compared to the medical community's ICD-9-CM codes, which describe the actual disease or injury. NANDA currently contains 167 approved diagnoses classified into nine domains. Each diagnosis consists of a label, definition, major and minor defining characteristics, and related factors.

An ICNP research and development project began in 1996 at São João College of Nursing in Porto, Portugal. Components of EHRs began appearing in Portugal during the 1990s. However, the autonomous dimension of nursing was invisible in those early systems. This was due, in part, to the difficulty of putting nursing content in the EHR. Clearly, concepts in the nursing domain needed to be articulated and formalized for inclusion in the EHR.

The purposes of this project were to (a) develop, with practicing nurses and using ICNP, the core concepts that describe their practice, in particular nursing diagnoses and nursing interventions, and (b) integrate core concepts of nursing in a nursing information model for the EHR.

The project began with exploring the description of nursing practice in Portugal. Nursing interventions are any treatment, based upon clinical judgment and knowledge, that a nurse performs to enhance patient outcomes (Dochterman & Bulechek, 2004). Consistent with Dochterman and Bulechek's definition, nursing regulations in Portugal assume that nursing interventions include nurse-initiated, physician-initiated, and other provider-initiated treatments. The regulations clearly state that a nurse-initiated treatment is an autonomous action initiated by the nurse in response to a nursing diagnosis, based on scientific rationale, and executed to benefit the client in a predictable way.

Meleis (2000) used the concept of transitions to describe the scope of nursing and its professional domain. The autonomous dimension of nursing thus encompasses professional interventions with people who are experiencing transitions with, for example, an illness, role change, or change in developmental state. The term *transitions* is not used within the Portuguese nursing community; however, transitions do occur. Today's transitions are reflected on the part of

Portuguese citizens in the need for self-care dependency situations, caregiver role challenges, and complex therapeutic regimes. These situations are well-suited for nursing care, including nursing diagnoses and autonomous nursing interventions. However, nursing practice in Portugal continues to be strongly oriented toward disease management. Basto (1998) reported a gap between theory-based nursing education and clinical practice anchored excessively in the management of signs and symptoms.

PROJECT IMPLEMENTATION
CONCEPT IDENTIFICATION

Following an initial action-research project, the São João College of Nursing formed the Nursing Information Systems Research Unit (NISRU) from which to launch this larger project. Nurses from three hospital units and three health centers were invited to participate in the discussion of their nursing practice model framework, to include their challenges in the reality of Portuguese health care. ICNP provided a common terminology for all participants. ICNP Alpha Version (ICN, 1996) was translated into Portuguese, and 8 hours of education about ICNP were provided to the nurse participants.

Nurses from these participating centers then worked to identify the core concepts for their nursing practice. The most frequent nursing phenomena (nursing diagnoses) in each care unit were identified, independent of the phenomena that were regularly used in their documentation. Nursing interventions were developed for each phenomenon, using the ICNP terminology. The nurse participants also reviewed applicable nursing literature to supplement the nursing phenomena and interventions identified in their work groups on the basis of their clinical practice.

EHR NURSING MODEL

The aims guiding the development of the EHR nursing model were (a) systematic, efficient documentation with minimal duplication, (b) referential integrity between the elements of nursing documentation, (c) natural language use and ICNP as the reference terminology, (d) inclusion of unit-specific common aspects of care, and (e) data collection and documentation throughout the patient's care episode for dynamic and meaningful care planning. The developers intended the model for use with either paper or electronic systems.

OUTCOMES ACHIEVED

The expertise of nurses in clinical practice provided the nursing phenomena and interventions that were most appropriate to their care settings. This met the assumption that nurses participating in the project would have a sense of ownership and would realize that their work resulted in substantive, valued contributions to the EHR. A major consequence of the project was that as nurses began to work with ICNP, they had the opportunity to truly reflect on their practice. Nurses talked together about what they actually were doing in their daily practice and how they would represent their practice using ICNP.

The project's five aims for the nursing model to be integrated with the EHR were achieved. The model was developed to facilitate pre-coordination of terms, pre-association of nursing diagnoses and nursing interventions, and the articulation between the natural language and the standardized language. In addition, the model supported the rules of association between nursing diagnoses and interventions; the organization of the nursing interventions to be implemented; and the rules of the referential integrity among the diagnoses, the status, the interventions, and the data resulting from the continuous observation of the patient. All of these outcomes contributed to an EHR that supported the nurses' practice, specifically in decision-making and workflow processes.

CHALLENGES AND OPPORTUNITIES

Implementing change in nursing practice is always a challenge. The researchers in Portugal found that nurses, in selecting concepts to represent their practice, thought differently from one another. For example, a patient with a stroke might represent *paresis* and *hypertension* to one nurse while the same patient might represent *self-care deficit* to another nurse. In developing EHRs, the consideration of these different ways of articulating the work of nursing is critical to achieving representation of all relevant nursing concepts.

Once the nursing model was implemented in the EHR for hospital settings, the project continued in two directions. One continuation phase covered the definition, development, and implementation of an infrastructure capable of adequate articulation and exchange of information between hospitals and health centers (Sousa, 2006). The efficient exchange of information between hospitals and health centers aimed to promote continuity of care across these settings.

The second continuation phase involved working with nurses in focus groups to develop a nursing data aggregation model to automatically produce health quality indicators in areas very sensitive to nursing care (Pereira, 2004). Those indicators, retrievable from the EHR, would reflect clinical nurses' own views on what constitutes nursing care quality.

ICNP Beta 2 Version was released in 2001, and ICNP Version 1.0 was released in 2005. Each version had to be translated into Portuguese to continue this work. Version 1.0 was a major revision of Beta 2, meaning that all users and researchers had to understand the new approach to application of the terminology (ICN, 2005).

The project has contributed to Portugal's work with ICNP. The Ordem dos Enfermeiros, the national nurses association in Portugal, has supported the translation of ICNP Version 1.0 and has sponsored a new initiative to promote national standards for nursing information system applications in Portugal. These standards will help ensure the quality of information systems used by nurses in Portugal.

LESSONS LEARNED

Nurses need to be involved in decisions involving the information systems they will use in their practice. Nurse participants asked, "How can we have worked in a setting for so long and these things have never been discussed before?" This project provided an opportunity for nurses to participate in EHR development throughout Portugal.

The work is never done. The work in Portugal to articulate the work of nursing began in the early 1990s and continues today. In addition to having great national impact on EHR development and using ICNP, Portugal serves as an exemplar to nursing groups around the world working toward EHRs that fully support nursing documentation and research.

RECOMMENDATIONS

Health information systems development and application is a long-term commitment. Nurses (clinicians, informatics experts, and researchers) need to be engaged in all levels of EHR development and implementation. The ICNP Programme works with nurses at local, national, and international levels to support the ongoing development of ICNP. The ICNP review process is used by nurses worldwide to recommend concept additions, modifications, or deletions. Nurses working collaboratively to advance ICNP may apply to become an ICN-Accredited Centre for ICNP Research and Development with concurrent membership in the ICNP Consortium.

REFERENCES

Basto M. (1998). Da intenção de mudar à mudança – Um caso de intervenção num grupo de enfermeiras, Rei dos livros, Lisboa.

Dochterman J.M. and Bulechek G. M. (Eds.) (2004). Nursing Interventions Classification (NIC). St Louis, MO: Mosby.

ICN. (1996). The International Classification for Nursing Practice A Unifying Framework. Geneva, Switzerland: International Council of Nurses.

ICN. (2005). The International Classification for Nursing Practice Version 1.0. Geneva, Switzerland: International Council of Nurses.

Meleis, A. (2000). Experiencing transitions: an emerging middle-range theory. Advances in Nursing Science, September, 23 (1): 12–28.

North American Nursing Diagnosis Association. (n.d.). *History & Historical Highlights 1973 Through 1998*. Retrieved 27 September 2007 from http://www.nanda.org/html/history1. html.

Pereira, F. (2004). Dos resumos mínimos de dados de enfermagem aos indicadores de ganhos em saúde sensíveis aos cuidados de enfermagem : o caminho percorrido; Ordem dos Enfermeiros; Suplemento don 13 (Jul. 2004), 13–21.

Sousa P. (2006). Sistema de partilha de informação de enfermagem entre contextos de saúde: um modelo explicativo. Formasau; Coimbra.

6

Global Standards and Certification

Mary Alexander, RN, CRNI, MA, CAE

Infusion therapy is ubiquitous regardless of the country where it is being administered. Patients in all countries are aware of intravenous (IV) catheters or have vascular access devices (VADs) inserted to receive their prescribed therapies, and they deserve to receive safe, quality infusion care. Outside of the United States (US), physicians have typically been the health-care professionals who have inserted the patients' VADs; however, more and more nurses are assuming that responsibility. Nurses have always been the providers involved with care, maintenance, and monitoring of the VADs.

Although infusion therapy has been recognized as a specialty nursing practice in the US for more than 60 years, many countries are just beginning to learn of its existence within the scope of professional nursing. Education specific to infusion therapy varies among and within countries. Consistent use of terminology and standardized practice may be minimal or nonexistent.

DESCRIPTION OF THE PROJECT

In 2005, I was invited to Mexico by PiSA Pharmaceuticals, a manufacturer of infusion-related products and solutions, to deliver lectures to Mexican physicians and nurses on integrating and applying standards of practice and guidelines to clinical practice. With a strong background as an infusion nurse and as the chief executive officer of the Infusion Nurses Society (INS), I was in a position to promote the benefits of an educated workforce delivering infusion care. INS is an international membership organization for the specialty practice of infusion nursing. The Society develops education programs, products, and services for infusion nurses and other health-care professionals who are involved in administering infusion care. INS has developed the *Infusion Nursing Standards of Practice*, a document that defines the scope of practice and educational requirements for nurses practicing infusion therapy. The *Standards* are based on evidence-based research and are to be applied in clinical practice regardless of the clinical setting in which care is delivered. This document gives a framework to organizations for creating their own policies and determining their criteria for the clinicians' competencies. With the complexity of patient conditions along the health-care continuum and advances in technology, it is imperative that nurses possess the knowledge and develop the skills to provide safe care.

During my travels in Mexico, it was clear that many of the Mexican nurses were interested in expanding their knowledge base relative to infusion nursing. They were beginning to understand that educating nurses on best practices of infusion care would be beneficial to the patient and the health-care system. In fact, in 1999 one group had already taken the first steps in developing a program that would be the basis for successful clinical outcomes for their infusion patients. At Hospital Angeles Pedregal in Mexico City, Mexico, part of the Grupo Angeles Healthcare System, protocols for care of central VADs were developed. This initiative was spearheaded by Ms. Guadalupe Ibarra, RN, MHA, Grupo Angeles' Director of Nursing. She was the leader and champion of this project, and a plan was created that would ultimately culminate in the first nursing course on infusion therapy in Mexico.

OUTCOMES ACHIEVED

Grupo Angeles' School of Health, supported by the University of Mexico, which is recognized by Mexico's Ministry of Education, developed an infusion program for nurses that would provide the knowledge and skills needed to deliver safe, standardized infusion care. In January 2007, the first class began the 10-week, 200-hour comprehensive course. It was based on the *Infusion Nursing Standards of Practice* and *Core Curriculum for Infusion Nursing*, with 40% of the program being in a didactic format, and the remaining 60% consisting of practical hands-on clinical experience. In collaboration with local public hospitals, the students were able to satisfy their clinical requirements.

On March 23, 2007, 21 nurses completed Mexico's first infusion therapy course. Class time gave them the ability to broaden their knowledge base of the specialty practice, while the clinical component allowed them to sharpen their technical expertise. This learning experience also increased the nurses' confidence about this critical component of patient care and stressed the importance of sharing their new knowledge and skills with their colleagues.

Unexpected Challenges And Opportunities

The opportunities outweigh any of the challenges that were encountered. As nurses we may be in different countries with different practices; however, we all have the same goal in mind—to deliver safe care to our patients. Since the inception of INS in 1973, the organization has developed fundamental infusion therapy programs that can be used in practice outside the US. Incorporating existing materials such as the *Infusion Nursing Standards of Practice* that are to be used in all practice settings allows the nurses to focus on other areas that need to be addressed rather than having to create their own original programs. Also, sharing this knowledge of the specialty increases chances that universal terminology and standardized care will be adopted in these foreign countries.

The main challenges include language barriers and comprehension of the medical terminology. When you are giving oral presentations or translating written materials, it is at times difficult to find the foreign equivalent for the English words. Also, it is necessary to ensure that any translations accurately reflect the content.

Lessons Learned

Although a program may be proposed, implementation may take time until all parties are comfortable that the content is accurate and the process is appropriate. Be prepared to review several phases of a program before a final version can be agreed on. Translating medical terminology and explaining clinical concepts in simple terms are necessary so that accuracy in the foreign language is achieved. Because this course was based on materials from INS, it was important that the organization have the opportunity to review the program content before its implementation.

Words of Wisdom

When making a change or trying to implement something new, identifying a champion who supports the initiative is imperative. Without Ms. Ibarra's leadership and vision, this first infusion course in Mexico may not have come to fruition at this time. Her knowledge of current clinical practice and the political infrastructure of the Mexican health-care system maximized the effectiveness of the process. Because INS did not have a physical presence in Mexico, it was helpful to let Grupo Angeles move forward at its own pace so that the appropriate channels would be followed and the course initiated.

To achieve success, start projects on a small scale so that outcomes can be realized. This first infusion course had 21 students enrolled. Evaluations of the course by the students and faculty will be helpful in making modifications that will enhance future programs. Sharing expertise and knowledge with our foreign colleagues is a rewarding experience. Our differences may be many; however, our objectives are similar as we seek to provide the best care that our patients deserve.

7

Network Weaving: A Story about Collegial Interest in the Teaching and Learning of Clinical Reasoning in Nursing

Daniel J. Pesut, PhD, RN, CS, FAAN
Ruth Anne Kuiper RN, PhD, CCRN
Carme Espinosa I. Fesnedo, RN, BSN, MSc

Edward Tufte (2006) in his book *Beautiful Evidence* suggests that the common analytic task in nearly all disciplines is to help people understand causality, make multivariate comparisons, examine relevant evidence, and assess the credibility of evidence and conclusions. Clinical reasoning involves knowledge and understanding of discipline-specific knowledge in addition to mastery of critical, creative systems, and complexity thinking skills. The art, science, and complexity of thinking that supports clinical reasoning include issues of structure, process, framing, action, strategy, outcomes, and clinical judgment. Essential elements of clinical reasoning include attention to beautiful evidence, structure, processes, and outcomes. As a result of many years of teaching experience, Daniel Pesut, one of the authors of this story, developed an innovative model of clinical reasoning and complementary teaching-learning strategies that departed from traditional ways to teach students the nursing process.

Nursing students spend countless hours completing care plans, or care maps, and faculty make judgments about students' clinical thinking through the evaluation of the nursing process documented on these teaching-learning artifacts. Little educational research evidence exists that supports the effectiveness of these artifacts on student learning or clinical reasoning skill acquisition. The Outcome Present State Test (OPT) Model (Pesut & Herman, 1992; 1998; 1999) of reflective clinical reasoning builds on the heritage of the nursing process and better fits contemporary needs for outcome specification and attention to clinical judgment. Dr. Pesut worked with a colleague, Dr. Ruth Anne Kuiper, on the development of her dissertation in self-regulated learning. Self-regulated learning is an important self-management process in learning how to think and reason.

The OPT model of reflective clinical reasoning is a meta-model of clinical reasoning that emphasizes reflection, outcome specification, and tests of judgment within the context of individual patient stories. The model advocates that clinicians concurrently consider relationships between and among competing diagnoses associated with a patient's nursing care needs. Such concurrent consideration enables one to reflect and reason and explain how the balancing and reinforcing loops and causal connections among the diagnoses influence each other. The relationships among diagnoses are mapped and represented in a thinking-reasoning tool called a Clinical Reasoning Web (CRW). As patterns and relationships among nursing care diagnoses are linked and connections explained what often emerges is a "keystone" issue that holds the system dynamics in place. A book about the model (Pesut & Herman, 1999) and several articles about implementation and evaluation of the model began to appear in the literature. Interestingly enough, nurses in Europe and the United Kingdom (UK) became curious about the model and wanted to learn more about it. One of the reasons people were curious was that the model seemed to accommodate and provide a structure for the use of emerging and developing nursing knowledge classification schemes like nursing diagnoses, nursing outcomes, and nursing interventions.

DESCRIPTION OF THE ANDORRA EXPERIENCE

Professor Carme Espinosa from Andorra, a member of the Associación Española de Nomenclatura, Taxonomia y Diagnóstica de Enfermería (AENTDE), contacted Dr. Pesut about his work with OPT. Professor Espinosa wanted to learn more about the model and invited Dr. Pesut to Valencia, Spain, to address a meeting of the AENTDE. After this initial visit, Dr. Pesut returned to Spain a second time and co-presented a workshop with Professor Espinosa about the use of the OPT Model of Clinical Reasoning to Spanish nurses. As a result of relationships developed across borders, Professor Espinosa visited the United States (U.S.) and worked more closely with Dr. Kuiper to learn how the OPT model was being implemented in undergraduate nursing programs in the U.S. Professor Espinosa visited with Dr. Kuiper in North Carolina and continued the collaboration and mutual learning described in the project. Professor Espinosa continues to modify and adapt the OPT model in her education program. She travels extensively throughout Europe and is actively diffusing the model in both education and practice settings.

In April of 2007, Dr. Pesut was invited to Amsterdam to present a keynote address at the Association for Common European Nursing Diagnoses, Interventions, and Outcomes (ACEN-

DIO) conference. In addition to the keynote address, Dr. Pesut and Professor Espinosa presented a tutorial on the use of OPT to an international and interdisciplinary group of colleagues
interested in nursing informatics and interdisciplinary communication.

The extensive use of the OPT model at an American nursing program was of interest to
Professor Espinosa. Because the OPT model was integrated throughout the curriculum at the
University of North Carolina (UNC) Wilmington, where Dr. Kuiper is a tenured associate professor, Dr. Kuiper organized a visit for Professor Espinosa to help her learn how the model was
used.

DESCRIPTION OF PROJECT

When Professor Espinosa came to the US, she spent about one week with Dr. Kuiper learning
about the implementation of the model and discussing the cognitive and metacognitive skills
that support clinical reasoning (Kuiper & Pesut, 2004). Dr. Kuiper explained how the model
was implemented in the curriculum at UNC Wilmington. In the nursing curriculum at UNC
Wilmington, clinical reasoning courses are taken by first semester junior-level nursing students.
Students are introduced to evidence-based practice, the research process, and clinical reasoning
strategies. The OPT model is delivered as a lecture and self-study module and applied through
use of case studies. Students are simultaneously enrolled in their first clinical nursing courses.
The OPT model is introduced in parts on a weekly basis. Students work toward completion of
OPT model worksheets that were developed to support the use of the model. Thereafter, the
OPT model is used in clinical nursing courses throughout the curriculum. Each course uses
the OPT model as a developmental step in reasoning about the nursing care needs of clients.
Examples of completed OPT models from each nursing course were reviewed and critiqued by
Professor Espinosa, which included completed worksheets from the areas of medical/surgical
nursing, home health nursing, psych/mental health nursing, chronic illness management, and
critical-care nursing.

Representative OPT model examples from each clinical area were shared and evaluated
for evidence of the structure, content, and process the students used to work through as they
developed clinical reasoning skills required to solve problems and make decisions in practice
situations. Strict adherence to the OPT model structure is required when completing these assignments in the American nursing curriculum. The entries in each section were evaluated by

the OPT model rating scale (Kautz, Kuiper, Pesut, Knight-Brown, & Daneker, 2005). In this program, clinical faculty share feedback with the students, affirming appropriate thinking strategies and suggesting areas that need improvement. Because the OPT model is used in the entire undergraduate nursing curriculum in the North Carolina program, the students are expert at the process by the final semester of the senior year.

As a result of the cross-cultural exchange and consultation, the greatest discrepancy discovered between the two educators was in the areas of adherence to standardized nursing language. According to Professor Espinosa, students she works with in Spain are required to pay particular attention to the details of nursing knowledge classifications and relationships between and among nursing diagnoses: definitions and classification (NANDA), nursing interventions (NIC), and nursing outcomes (NOC) systems. While the OPT model supports a structure to accommodate the use of NANDA, NIC, and NOC language, many faculty in the U.S. program have not totally adopted the use of standardized languages. Representation and classification of nursing knowledge is an important professional issue. The evolution and development of standardized nursing language has included a systematic program of research over the past 32 years, resulting in significant advancements in nursing knowledge work. Standardized nursing language exists to represent relationships between and among nursing diagnoses, interventions, and outcomes. When these languages are used to structure nursing information systems in hospitals and other health-care organizations, nursing care, activities, interventions, and achievement of nursing-sensitive outcomes are evident.

It is imperative that educators anticipate the adoption and dispersion of standardized nursing language and become more intentional about teaching and using a clinical vocabulary that supports students' clinical reasoning about patient care needs, nursing solutions, and nursing interventions.

With respect to the application in Andorra, this cultural or across the border difference was striking. Europeans are much more advanced in the use of informatics and standardized languages than are their U.S.-based counterparts. In contrast, the reflective process that supports development of clinical reasoning was more explicit at the American campus because of the use of structured journaling and self-regulated learning prompts that provided a stimulus for student thinking and responding. Such self-regulated learning prompts help students determine which thinking skill to revisit and, in doing so, promote the memory and habit of thinking and reflecting.

After sharing the programmatic examples, Professor Espinosa spent a day in a critical-care clinical area to shadow nursing faculty who were supervising students and observe the implementation of the OPT model by the students and the debriefing students received in one-on-one conferences. Professor Espinosa also witnessed how the model was used during human patient simulation experiences with a group of students who used the OPT model worksheets as a scenario debriefing activity.

The self-study modules used to introduce students to the model by both professors were compared, contrasted, and evaluated. This exercise revealed tremendous similarities in how the OPT model is disseminated to faculty and students across the two countries. The differences discovered were primarily related to cultural nuances and educator styles and preferences. The adoption of educational pedagogies was similar between cultures. The theoretical principles that supported the teaching and learning effort associated with use of the OPT model appeared to be the same.

Outcomes

Some outcomes to date have included

1. Presentations at two Spanish Nursing Diagnosis Conferences.

2. An invitation to present at the 2007 ACENDIO Conference.

3. A published interview in Spanish on "Clinical Reasoning in Nursing and the OPT Model."

4. An international exchange between an American educator, Dr. Kuiper, and European educator, Professor Espinosa, to share ideas and experiences surrounding implementation of the OPT model of clinical reasoning and to learn and understand the history of pedagogical strengths and barriers from a cross-cultural perspectives. See Table P-7.1.

TABLE P-7.1. NEW DIAGNOSES REVIEW PROCESS.

New diagnoses go through *a full review process*, which includes the following steps

1. Posting on the NANDA-I web site

2. Review of submission by the primary reviewer

3. Primary reviewer works with submitter to address changes that need to be made

4. Submission is forwarded to full Diagnosis Development Committee (DDC) for review.

5. DDC recommends one of the following:

    a. Approve with no recommendations

    b. Approve pending follow-through with recommendations (most frequent DDC decision)

    c. Disapprove

6. The primary reviewer forwards the DDC recommendations to the submitter and works with the submitter to make the recommended changes.

7. Submissions approved by the DDC are presented and discussed at the biennial conference in order to invite extended member input. Recommendations from the forums are reviewed with the submitter and by the DDC.

8. The submission is then forwarded to the NANDA International Board of Directors for final approval. Diagnoses accepted at the 2.1 level of development will be incorporated into both the NANDA-I Taxonomy II and the NNN Taxonomy of Nursing Practice, and published in the next edition of *NANDA-I Nursing Diagnoses: Definitions & Classification.*

UNEXPECTED CHALLENGES

Differences in language proved to be a challenge and an opportunity. Communicating across times zones and countries was also a challenge. Although sometimes it is difficult because of language restraints, the fact is that sharing transcultural experiences is an excellent way of improving knowledge. From the point of view of Professor Espinosa, the experience was a challenge from the beginning. The implementation of the OPT model was a risky decision because at the time no other nursing school in neighboring European countries was using the model. But on another hand that was an opportunity to see that the differences between what was happening in terms of teaching and learning clinical reasoning in the US and Andorra were not so big.

The opportunity to influence and learn from colleagues across the globe proved to be very interesting. For example, it is clear that colleagues in the European countries are far more advanced in their use and understanding of nursing informatics and nursing diagnoses than colleagues in the US. Also, it is interesting to note that nursing information systems in European countries are being standardized and in many cases supported and mandated by government agencies. Funds and resources exist to implement nursing information systems so that nursing diagnoses, interventions, and outcomes might be captured and analyzed to better understand nursing contributions to the health-care enterprise.

Lessons Learned

Curiosity about nursing colleagues work is an invitation for connection and collaboration. Professor Espinosa contacted Dr. Pesut personally to inquire about his work and the OPT model. The relationship established across borders and the co-commitment to the scholarship of teaching and learning developed through time.

Connecting with one colleague gives one access to a network of colleagues. As a result of Professor Espinosa's initiative in contacting Dr. Pesut, he in turn connected her with others who were using and experimenting with the OPT model. This "closing the triangle" is a network weaving strategy. It happens when two people connect and then invite a third or more to relate in a social network. Closing the triangle is a key factor in creating and evolving "smart networks." People who do the connecting are called "network weavers." Holley and Krebs (2007) describe how to build smart communities through network weaving. Professor Espinosa continues to be a "network weaver" bringing information to nurses through out Spain and Europe about the OPT model.

Words of Wisdom

Take advantage of collegial networks. In today's health-care environment, nursing professionals from different sectors and from different countries usually meet at international conferences. That is a good opportunity to meet, greet, connect, and plan periodic follow-up encounters with those who want to share experiences and knowledge. Professionals from smaller countries or smaller universities should have the courage to seek out the work of colleagues that they believe is aligned with their professional interests. Be curious and reach out to connect with those people as most are willing to respond, and are delighted to share their work in hopes that the works will be used, diffused and enhanced. Remember that everybody has something to teach and something to learn; take advantage of the opportunities through international network weaving.

REFERENCES AND RESOURCES

Holley, J. & Krebs, V.. Building smart communities through network weaving. Retrieved March 1, 2007 at http://www.orgnet.com/BuildingNetworks.pdf

Kautz, D., Kuiper, R., Pesut, D., Knight-Brown, P., & Daneker, D. (2005). Promoting Clinical Reasoning in Undergraduate Nursing Students: Application and Evaluation of the Outcome Present State Test (OPT) Model of Clinical Reasoning, *International Journal of Nursing Education Scholarship*: Vol. 2, No. 1. Retrieved 27 September 2007 from http://www.bepress.com/ijnes/vol2/iss1/art1/.

Kuiper, R. & Pesut, D. (2004). Promoting cognitive and metacognitive reflective learning skills in nursing practice: Self-regulated learning theory. *Journal of Advanced Nursing*, 45 (4), 381–391.

Pesut, D. & Herman, J. (1999). *Clinical reasoning: The art and science of critical and creative thinking*. New York: Delmar Publishers.

Pesut, D. & Herman, J. (1998). OPT: Transformation of the Nursing Process for contemporary practice. *Nursing Outlook,* 46: 29–36.

Pesut, D. J. & Herman, J. (1992). Metacognitive skills in diagnostic reasoning: Making the implicit explicit. *Nursing Diagnosis*, 3(4), 148–154.

8

MIGRATION

CLARITA D. CURATO, RN, MAN, EdD

MA. KATHERINE O. JIONGCO, RN, BSN

JO ELLEN KOERNER, PhD, RN, FAAN

Migration is the evolutionary urge of life. Found in every species on the planet, it is the outcome of a relentless curiosity that invites us to probe the edges of our everyday world and see what lies beyond. Because curiosity is our birthright, migration from the safe sanctuary of our childhood home into the larger world is the first initiating step in the outward direction. For many of us it stops somewhere within the borders of our homeland. But for the pilgrims and pioneers within our clan, the world calls further.

Nursing is a universal phenomenon. While the culture and language vary by reflecting the geography in which we reside, the human body is of one form. The core essence of human wants and needs, as well as dreams and delights, is one, and at the end of the day, we are one.

Converging sociopolitical changes, technological interventions, and economic realities are altering the provision of health-care services globally. Newer structures and relationships continue to emerge, requiring practices and processes different from those used in the past. Nursing is at the crossroads, facing shortages of unparalleled proportion at a time when society is experiencing health-care challenges of great magnitude. This growing global shortage is prompting a mass migration of nursing professionals around the world. Caring and commerce meet at this intersection, requiring an ethical stance so that the health-care needs of the world are maintained.

A socially responsible model of nurse migration has been created through a business-service partnership between the United States (US) and the Philippines. It was designed to strengthen the education and competency of nurses on both sides of the globe, enhancing the care for all.

THE PHILIPPINES

The Philippines, also known as the *Pearl of the Orient* and the *Island of the Smiles*, is the world's second largest archipelago. Manila, the capital, covers a land area of 300,000 square kilometers with a population of nearly 87 million. English is one of the official languages; the local language has multiple dialects, but Tagalog is the most popular. The literacy rate is 94%. Religions practiced by the people include Roman Catholicism (82%), Iglesia ni Cristo and other Christian denominations (9%), Islam (5%), and other religions (4%).

The people's hard work, resiliency, and patriotism that have helped the nation triumph over the domestic and global, political, and economic challenges it continues to face (U.S. Library of Congress, 1991).

Principles and Relationships: Vertical Integration Model

Because nursing is a universal phenomenon, the basic education and experience of a nurse is global in nature. A credentialing transfer can be achieved by meeting the requisite licensure and immigration requirements. Movement in the global market is limited, primarily, by language, cultural norms, and clinical experience barriers. The technical complexity and professional autonomy in U.S. practice is not found everywhere. Until now, only the language barrier has been addressed. The establishment of a vertical integration model, focused on expansion of basic core competencies through skill enhancement, will remove the last barriers to a truly universal professional. Global Resources for Outsourced Workers, Inc. (GROW), is this agent of transformation.

GROW

GROW was founded in 2002 by entrepreneurial visionaries who had dreamed of introducing global employment opportunities for many Filipinos who have the heart, skills, and passion to contribute in a productive and positive way. This dream is fueled by the understanding that Filipinos are and will continue to be a positive force for change throughout the world. Within the health-care sphere, it is a well known fact that Filipinos excel as nurses and general caregivers.

Since the mid 1990s, major U.S. hospitals and other nursing institutions around the globe have raised a quiet clamor to see the international nurse recruitment industry elevate its standards in the preparation and delivery of qualified nursing professionals to work in advanced health-care economies. GROW has met this need by recruiting, preparing, and building a significant supply of nurses who meet international standards of competency, as well as capably adjust to the rigors brought about by international nursing mobility. A market leader, GROW has created a vertically integrated human resources supply chain model that takes advantage of affiliated relationships among nursing schools, hospitals, and professional development and review centers in the Philippine that are bound together via common shareholder ownership. This is further reinforced through demonstrated service expertise in the areas of U.S. immigration and relocation support.

The vertical integrated infrastructure provides Filipino nurses access to world-class learning systems and technologies that are needed by nurses to acquire minimum competencies to function as a U.S. registered nurse.

Adventist HealthCare

In 2004, GROW entered into a strategic relationship with one of the leading U.S. health-care systems, Adventist HealthCare (AHC) based out of Rockville, Maryland.

Washington Adventist Hospital, the flagship of AHC, was founded by the Seventh-Day Adventist Church in 1907. Since its beginning, the hospital has reflected the church's beliefs that physical, mental, and spiritual health care are essential components of a person's well-being. In 1999 Washington Adventist Hospital was named one of America's "Top 100 Interventional Cardiovascular Programs" by Solucient, formerly known as HCIA, a leading national independent health-care information company. Today, Adventist HealthCare is a comprehensive network of hospitals, nursing and rehabilitation centers, home health-care agencies, and other specialized health-care services. Recognizing that both the internal and external populations that the hospital serves represent many cultures and languages, Adventist currently has employees who can translate more than 24 different languages and dialects, including sign language. This culturally sensitive philosophy prompted a relationship with GROW, Inc. The partnership has resulted in the establishment of a U.S.-based company called GROW Health-care (GHC), which is wholly owned by AHC.

GHC works with various health-care institutions to consider international recruitment as a viable supplemental strategy to address nursing workforce shortages and offers a turnkey approach to recruitment that insulates client hospitals from the associated risks inherent in the processing of internationally educated nurses for employment in the US.

DE LOS SANTOS COLLEGE OF NURSING AND SYSTEMS TECHNOLOGY, INC.

Systems Technology Incorporated (STI), the parent company of GROW, operates the largest network of information technology (IT) and nursing schools in the Philippines. More than 100 colleges and education centers belong to the STI Education Network, including 21 colleges of nursing, the oldest one being the De Los Santos-STI College of Health Professions (DLS-STI).

The De Los Santos College was established and recognized by the education department in 1975 as part of the expanding services of the De Los Santos Medical Center to the Filipino community. The school opened its college of nursing with only 65 students; current applicants represent the country's finest students with scores of 95% in their exams. Through diligence and careful management, the college has increased its student population to 300 annually.

Since its opening in 1975, the De Los Santos School of Nursing has always been a separate institution from the hospital. A September 2002 merger between the college and STI further facilitated growth. Thus, the name De Los Santos-STI College of Health Professions, Inc., was established. To this date, the partnership has created an environment responsive to the national goals of empowering people with information and communications technology enhanced quality health-care education to make them globally competitive and employable.

GROW, in partnership with DLS-STI and Adventist, believe that education is the strongest molding force in the holistic development of an individual. Their mission is as follows:

> Recruit highly qualified and culturally-prepared professionals to meet the temporary and permanent staffing needs of companies across the globe. We ensure timely deployment of globally-competitive professionals to our clients by way of meticulous and intelligent recruitment, pre-qualification and selection coupled with the utilization of the latest technologies. (GROW, n.d.)

Meaning and merit are measured through academic excellence, nationalism, love of God, discipline, respect for humanity, and promotion of a just and peaceful society.

PARTNERSHIP PROCESSES

The criteria for recruiting, selecting, and processing of nurses for GROW depends on the interplay of three key timelines, which are seen in Table P-8.1.

TABLE P-8.1.   KEY FACTORS

(1) Experiential Timeline

- GROW recruits nurses who have the potential to be top performers when they begin work at U.S. hospitals.

- Emphasis is on the quality of clinical nursing practice gained while the nurse is still in the country.

- GROW applies an in-depth screening during a one-on-one interview with the nurses:

  - Nurse Academic Characteristics involve nurse level of education and number of years in the nursing practice

  - Patient Characteristics involve acuity/severity of illness, stage of treatment process, and functional capacity

  - Organizational Characteristic involves type of clinical unit, nurse-to-patient ratio, and shift duration

  - Acceptance and Caring discusses the ability of the nurse to respect the rights of all people regardless of age, religious belief, status, and sexual orientation

  - Eagerness to Learn is about the nurse's motivation to keep up with nursing trends and to value life-long learning

  - Confidence shows the ability to handle crisis and everyday challenges in a positive, proficient, and compassionate way

  - Determination deals with the determination to succeed and be a good nurse

- The clinical experience, nursing skills, personality, and goals are taken into consideration, assuring a match between the nurse and the hospital requirement.

(2) Credentialing Timeline

- Emigrant nurses are expected to secure their nursing licensure before they start employment with the hospital.

- For internationally educated nurses, there is a need to identify the state of initial licensure; under a nursing registry, it is not always immediately known in what state the nurse will be employed. It is important, therefore, that the state of licensure allows for endorsement to the state where the nurse will ultimately work.

- Ensure education equivalency:

  - Internationally educated nurses should, at a minimum, have passed either the Commission on Graduates of Foreign Nursing Schools (CGFNS) exam or the National Council Licensure EXamination-Registered Nurse (NCLEX-RN) test.

  - To confirm the applicant has a level of competency in oral and written English, the nurse has to pass Test of English as a Foreign Language (TOEFL) and Test of Spoken English (TSE) or International English Language Test System (IELTS).

TABLE P-8.1.   KEY FACTORS (CONTINUED)

(3) Immigration Timeline

- This is the most unpredictable.

- Nurses who have passed and secured their CGFNS certificates or passed NCLEX are in the best position to begin the immigration paperwork.

- U.S. immigration laws are among the most rigid in the world.

- Immigration reform in the US is a complex issue, resulting in extreme delays in allowing foreign-educated nurses to come to the US to pursue nursing employment.

- Visa caps exist for many employment-based petitions, resulting in massive delays to bring in nurse workers. While on average it takes 12-14 months to process an immigrant visa for nurses, U.S. visa retrogression will most likely extend this out further by at least 6 months. Box P-8.1 provides an overview of obtaining a Visa screen certificate.

BOX P-8.1.   OBTAINING A VISA SCREEN CERTIFICATE.

U.S. Immigration law requires that health-care professionals (except physicians) qualified outside the United States complete a screening program to qualify for certain U.S. working visas (immigrant or working visa). The Visa Screen, also known as Visa Credentials Assessment, enables healthcare workers to meet this requirement by verifying and evaluating their credentials to ensure compliance with the government's minimum eligibility standards.

Visa Screen is administered by the International Commission on Healthcare Professions (ICHP), which is a division of Commission on Graduates of Foreign Nursing Schools (CGFNS). This certification authenticates that the foreign national's education, license, training, and experience are comparable to that of a U.S. health-care professional.

This certificate is presented to a U.S. consulate office as part of the application process of an occupational visa.

GROW partnerships are uniquely situated to support the progress of GROW nurses across the three key timelines. The vertical integrated model serves as the platform that nurses can tap to help them achieve each of these timelines, with the ultimate objective of having a licensed, productive, and capable nurse ready to assume work in the US.

CHALLENGES

Challenges to migrating from one country to another extend beyond the education/certification realm. Other issues that confront the nurse moving across borders include cross-cultural role and gender issues, language differences, and advanced technology.

CROSS-CULTURAL ISSUES

The core culture of the Filipino population is one of caring for others. Many Filipinos choose to remain within the borders of the old traditions, which makes it challenging to become multi-cultural. For example, Filipinos possess a value of respect for authority, making them non-confrontational and less self-confident in asserting personal views. Filipino culture believes in the authority of men over women and the superiority of physicians over nurses. Rather than be assertive, Filipinos prefer to blend into the background. Because they are unfamiliar with diverse cultural working conditions, Filipino nurses need to be familiarized with local cultures to ensure adaptation within those settings.

LANGUAGE DIFFERENCES

The use of slang and local accents creates comprehension challenges. Translation is often delayed, slowing the response time, and paraphrasing does not always allow the nurse to fully express the totality of their thoughts. The challenges of language differences, coupled with a personality that will defer, may give an impression about the knowledge and capability of the nurse that is inaccurate.

ADVANCED TECHNOLOGY

Working with modern equipment and disposable supplies is a new experience for some nurses. Reuse of medical supplies is common in the Philippines. Also, many of the "technologies" are portable pumps and devices that are taken to the patient bedside only when needed. The complexity of the human-technology interface is a great challenge for many who come to the US.

Only 30% of all Filipinos own a car, and the presence of computers and handheld devices is also minimal. While cybercafes are making a presence in the country, it is still not in the lives of the majority. Cell phones, on the other hand, are everywhere, and text messaging is a primary form of communication, especially amongst the younger generations.

OUTCOMES AND SUSTAINABILITY

A robust collection of businesses and services, linked together, create an ecosystem that supports and enhances the resource pool of nurses for global deployment and the quality of healthcare for the Philippines.

- Academic institutions, such as De Los Santos School of Nursing, offer the foundational education for an RN pool for global work.

- Training hospitals, such as De Los Santos Hospital and MegaClinic, offer clinical experiences for students. A continuing challenge is the maintenance of a highly skilled workforce as many RNs get the requisite competency and leave for other parts of the world. Modernizing the training laboratories in the hospital setting would enhance care for all.

- Support programs, such as the Universal Worker Training Center, provide English as Second Language training along with preparation courses. The addition of simulation-based training would further enhance the student capacity for the center and standardized professional development for the RN.

- Specialty health services, such as the Manila Adventist Medical Center and Children's Hospital, offer specific and complex patient populations leading to advanced practice, faculty, and staff development for specialty practice and certification. Enhancing the technology to support the care requirements would increase RN exposure to technologies routinely used in the US.

- Access to global employment, such as GROW, Inc., offers competent RNs deployment opportunities for direct placement into overseas facilities. It also places these RNs into registry programs that guarantee immediate employment. Resolving the immigration issues in the US would lift the retrogression barrier to movement across the borders.

- U.S.-based educational partners, such as Adventist Columbia Union College, offer cross-cultural training programs to facilitate advanced education for faculty and clinical leaders. It could also offer clinical specialty programs leading to specialty certification and care of complex patient populations in the Philippines.

GOING FORWARD

As in all other parts of the world, in the Philippines nurses have a deep desire to embrace the profession as a vocation as initiated by Florence Nightingale, notwithstanding the financial opportunities that are offered from all corners of the globe. As the shortage intensifies, it is critical for the profession to remain rooted in the values of service and caring.

Partnership has a robust quality and capacity that is not possible for any single entity to achieve. The vertical integration model with GROW has created a borderless platform where any nurse wanting to gain access to world-class training, education, and practices can tap from an abundant repository of tools and services.

The greater adoption of web-based content will help bring knowledge literally to the palm of every nurse wanting to hone his or her skills. The model serves as the tapestry whereby the collective experience in delivering quality nursing care will be within reach of every nursing professional. And a competent, mobile, and compassionate nursing workforce will provide quality care to society on a global scale.

REFERENCES

GROW, Inc. (n.d.). About us. Retrieved 3 October 2007 from http://www.growinc.net/about. php.

U.S. Library of Congress, Country Study Philippines, 1991-1999 Philippine Statistical Yearbook, National Statistical Coordination Board.

The authors acknowledge the assistance of Raymond L. Cantane, GROW, Inc.

Part VI

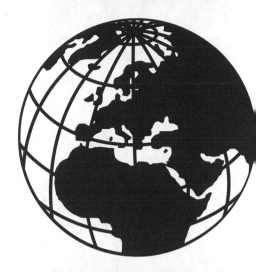

EDUCATIONAL
SUCCESS STORIES

When we address international partnerships in nursing, we immediately recognize that each of us is at once both student and teacher. Here, a dynamic group of global nursing leaders takes us through a series of documented successes that address all aspects of nursing, from basic educational preparation to advanced practice and doctoral education. From the classroom to the cruise ship, from the desert to the mission, education prevails. Through their initiatives, they have created a cadre of nurse leaders and educators for this century and beyond. Enjoy their stories and their experiences, and make them your own.

1

BUILDING A COMMUNITY OF NEW SCHOLARS

RITA M. CARTY, PHD, RN, FAAN

Saudi Arabia, not unlike other countries in the world is experiencing a nursing shortage. What distinguishes the Saudi Arabian shortage is the acute shortage of Saudi nurses prepared in Saudi Arabia. For many years most nursing positions, especially leadership positions, have been filled by expatriate nurses. Nurses from the Philippines and Egypt provide most of the bedside nursing, while administrators, managers, and educators have been recruited from the United States (US), Canada, the United Kingdom (UK), Australia, and New Zealand.

These factors combined to create a desire to prepare more Saudi nurses both within the country of Saudi Arabia and in educational programs in other countries to meet the nursing shortages needs in Saudi Arabia.

In the mid 1990s, a professional nursing education program was initiated between the Kingdom of Saudi Arabia and George Mason University, College of Nursing and Health Science in Fairfax, Virginia, US. The program was a collaborative education model with the purpose of building a community of new professionals in nursing who would also advance to be leaders, educators, administrators, and ultimately scholars in their own country. It was proposed that the actual practice, leadership, education, and research skills of the select groups would elevate the delivery of quality health care for the people of Saudi Arabia. This success story addresses the process and outcomes of 10 years of collaboration, knowledge, and resources incorporated into this international education program in nursing.

PROJECT DESCRIPTION

In 1995, the Saudi-US University Project (SUSUP) was initiated by collaboration between King Faisal Specialist Hospital and Research Center (KFSH&RC) in the Kingdom of Saudi Arabia and several US universities. The George Mason University College of Nursing and Health Science (GMU-CNHS) was the nursing participant in this project tasked to prepare highly qualified and competent Saudi bedside nurses who ultimately would become nurse leaders, educators, administrators, and new scholars. The program started in May 1995 with an approved budget of $1.3 million under SUSUP. Initially 12 male Saudi students who held a degree in science were selected to attend an accelerated baccalaureate of nursing (BSN) program at GMU-CNHS. A process was established for continued input and feedback between GMU-CNHS and KFSH&RC by real-time TV conferences, phone conferences, fax, and onsite visits to Saudi Arabia by GMU-CNHS faculty and to the US by administrators and educators from KFSH&RC. As a result of this collaboration, consultation input, and feedback, plus a strong curriculum and unique teaching strategies, 11 of the original 12 students completed the program and returned to Saudi Arabia.

Due to a life-threatening illness of Saudi Arabia's king the SUSUP project was put on hold. A 4-year period of non-funding then occurred. During this time several of the students from the original group pursued graduate education at GMU-CNHS. The program was funded again in 2000 by Prince Bandar bin Sultan with a budget of $1.8 million. This phase of the project was a continuation of the collaborative project between GMU-CNHS and KFSH&RC, plus two additional Saudi institutions: Saudi Arabia National Guard Hospital (SANG) and the Ministry of Aviation and Defense Hospital (MODA). The project concluded in 2005 with the graduation of the final group of students. The final group of students attended in 3 cohorts composed of 18 males and 7 females. In addition to science backgrounds, students with degrees in related fields were admitted. Two of the students in this phase did not complete the program for personal reasons.

OUTCOMES ACHIEVED

Over a 10-year period a total of 34 students, 27 males and 7 females, completed the program and earned baccalaureate degrees in nursing. Of this group, five have now completed doctoral degrees (PhD) in nursing, six have completed master's degree programs in nursing, and seven more are currently enrolled in nursing master's degree programs. All the graduates not currently in educational programs are practicing their profession in Saudi Arabia with the exception of one student who has completed medical school. Of those practicing, three are nursing administrators in large health-care facilities. Several are nurse managers on hospital units, and one is in medical records. The PhD graduates are achieving recognition as leaders and new scholars.

Lessons Learned

Although, much was learned by both the university and the sending agencies, the program also yielded many positive collaborative relationships. Consideration of international education, the role of culture in learning, and how to work together to achieve positive outcomes were the fabrics that ran throughout the 10 years.

Unexpected Challenges And Opportunities

By using graduating grade point average (GPA) as a benchmark we encountered some interesting and unexpected challenges. Either a Test of English as a Foreign Language (TOEFL) or English Language Institute (ELI) verification was required for admission but did not correlate with the graduating GPA. A higher admission GPA meant a higher graduating GPA. However, the project faculty found that no relationship existed between GPA, ELI, TOEFL, age, or number of children that any individual student had, which were common factors between all students. This finding is somewhat puzzling in regards to TOEFL or ELI, as experience clearly identified language skills as a challenge for these students' success. Language preparation should begin in the student's country before admission to intense academic programs in this country. Clearly the ELI program that the grant provided for on both a group and an individual basis made the difference with these students.

All male students had higher graduating GPA mean scores than the female students. In a predominately female profession such as nursing, and considering that these male students in many cases might have preferred another career, it is rewarding that the men had such high academic achievement. Academic achievement may reflect cultural influence. An expected outcome was that those students with science backgrounds would do better than those with backgrounds in the humanities. The project originally required all students to have science backgrounds, but when difficulty recruiting students who matched all admission requirements arose, this requirement was relaxed. However, a background in science was found to mean more success for this accelerated program and would be recommended for any future programs.

Married students with family in the US had a higher graduating GPA than single students. This was true for both male and female students. This was not an expected finding. In fact, the project faculty had encouraged students to come to the US without their family so as to have more time to study. It quickly became evident that married students both wanted and needed their families with them.

A strongly held belief of the project faculty was that students who had prior work experience in health-care settings, regardless of the nature of the experience, would be more successful than students without health care experience. Program evaluation indicated that when considering total student population, students without health care experience achieved a higher graduating GPA than those with health care experiences. However, male students with prior health care experiences scored a bit higher than males without health care experience and higher than female participants, all of whom had prior health care experience. Given the intensity and unfamiliarity of the Saudi students' nursing education in the US, it is possible that any prior health care experience they may have is so different as to be irrelevant to their US experience as nursing students. As a result, a background in health care may, at best, have limited impact on the students' success.

On admission, students were asked to articulate goals for a career in nursing, although at the time of admission the goals that the students listed were often fairly basic, such as "help sick people" and "work with the doctor." Even so, again using graduating GPA as a benchmark, those students who had at least a basic idea of what a career in nursing might entailed achieved higher graduating GPAs than the students who could not articulate goals.

Another surprise for the project faculty was that age was not significant in regard to success. It was thought that the younger students would be more successful. This did not prove to be true.

WORDS OF WISDOM

In light of the severe and deepening global nursing workforce shortage, many countries around the world are seeking ways to upgrade and increase the supply of qualified nurses within their own borders. This project offers a collaborative model, which had much success and contributed to the development of nursing practitioners, leaders, and new scholars who are improving the quality of health care to the people of Saudi Arabia now and in the future.

2

A UNIQUE SERVICE-EDUCATION PARTNERSHIP TO ADVANCE NURSING IN SAUDI ARABIA

LINDA LUNA, RN, PHD
SAWSAN ABDUL SALAM MAJALI, PHD, MSN, BSC, RN

In August 2002, a collaborative effort between Dar Al Hekma College and the King Faisal Specialist Hospital and Research Center in Jeddah, Saudi Arabia, was announced. The aim of the project was to develop and launch a new school of nursing in the western region of the country. This was a significant event because previous attempts to establish a nursing program in this region had failed. Many months of intense negotiation and planning preceded the announcement. These planning efforts had produced a shared vision and philosophy, an implementation plan, and specific strategies that formalized the resources and expertise that both organizations would contribute and share as part of this agreement. The new nursing program was a unique model of a nursing service/nursing education partnership aimed at building nursing capacity and ensuring an adequate supply of highly qualified nurses to meet the health care needs of the people of Saudi Arabia. The collaborative effort was a mutual understanding in that the hospital and the college were equal partners sharing in staff recruitment, teaching, and clinical training, with each organization contributing the types of resources (library, classrooms, laboratories, preceptors) needed to make the program a success.

The motivating factors for the two organizations to enter into an agreement to develop a nursing program were multifaceted. Like most countries in the world, the Kingdom of Saudi Arabia suffers from a shortage of nurses. Since the beginning of modern health care in Saudi Arabia in the 1950s, most nurses have been non-Saudi expatriates. In fact, only 26.6% of all nurses employed in the country today represent the national culture, with the majority prepared at the technical level and only 3% at the baccalaureate level (The Kingdom of Saudi Arabia Ministry of Health, 2006). For some time, the negative image of nursing as a profession failed to attract sufficient numbers to allow the country to become less dependent on recruitment of foreign nurses. Young women in Saudi Arabia traditionally were not encouraged to work outside the home and thereby faced complexities in both professional and personal decision making not experienced by most western women. In addition, young men are not guided toward seeking careers in nursing. The Ministry of Health (MOH) mandates that baccalaureate nursing programs in Saudi Arabia do not admit men, so men interested in pursuing nursing at the baccalaureate level must go outside of the kingdom.

A critical area of concern identified by the Saudi government is that nurses who provide health-care services to Saudi citizens should speak the language (Arabic) of the patient and understand the culture and religion. Therefore, a major push to "Saudi-ize" the nursing workforce has gained widespread endorsement in recent years. With a global nursing shortage looming on the horizon, continuing the high level of dependence on recruitment of foreign nurses was clearly not an effective or efficient strategy; Saudi Arabia needed to think about "growing their own." From a service perspective, many felt that having Saudi nurses provide care for the Saudi population would facilitate communication, improve patient outcomes, and reduce cultural conflict. From an academic perspective, developing a school of nursing was a strategic decision in supporting the college's social responsibility, as well as making major attempts at changing the negative image and status of nursing in the kingdom.

DESCRIPTION OF THE DEVELOPMENTAL PROCESS AND STRUCTURE OF THE SCHOOL

In 2000, King Faisal Specialist Hospital and Research Center opened in Jeddah as a sister institution to the flagship hospital in Riyadh. Within the first year, 600 nurses had been recruited for employment from some 40 countries around the world. By the end of the second year, the facility was recognized as providing health care of the highest quality and was accredited by Joint Commission International Accreditation (JCIA). After 9/11 and the exodus of a significant number of expatriate nurses from the kingdom, the importance of nursing resources became even more apparent to executive leaders. What had been envisioned in the months prior to the establishment of the program began to take shape as an important imperative for the future of health care in Saudi Arabia.

Dar Al Hekma is the first private non-profit college for women in the kingdom. Established in 1999, the program grew out of a collaborative effort between Texas International Education Consortium and education experts from the kingdom and western region of Saudi

Arabia. A lengthy collaboration resulted in 32 documents that served as the basis of the establishment of the college.

The college began with three programs—management of information systems, special education, and interior design. In 2002, nursing and graphic design programs were added. The purpose of the bachelor of science degree in nursing program is to prepare female nurses to meet the challenges of nursing practice in an ever-changing and increasingly complex world of health care. In developing the baccalaureate-level curriculum, representatives of Dar Al Hekma and King Faisal Specialist Hospital, as well as consultants from King Abdul Azziz University nursing faculty, embraced an overarching belief that nursing education that is collaborative in nature between academic and service settings can prepare students to survive the "real work world experience." After several curriculum drafts, final approval from the Ministry of Higher Education came in March 2004.

OUTCOMES ACHIEVED

From the beginning, recruitment of students and faculty was ongoing through a variety of means—announcements via school visits; college fairs; web sites; advertisements in local, national, and international print media; and word of mouth. In a strategic move to provide stability and continuity of the program, four Saudi nurses have been sponsored for graduate scholarships abroad to complete master's and doctoral degrees. Because of a shortage of qualified local faculty, the college recruits faculty from abroad for all programs. The working environment of the college includes comfortable classrooms with state-of-the-art educational equipment, computer laboratories, library facilities, and clinical learning laboratories. Faculty are supported to attend workshops and conferences both locally and abroad.

In 2004, the first International Nursing Conference was co-sponsored by King Faisal Specialist Hospital and Dar Al Hekma college. For many of the students, this was their first professional nursing conference and they assisted in registration, preparing booklets and conference bags, and in announcing speakers. In November 2005, the Evidence-Based Nursing Made Easy for Bedside Nurses conference was organized collaboratively between the hospital and the college as a follow-up to recommendations of the first nursing conference. The aim was to have nurses become comfortable in reading and applying research findings to nursing practice. Again, nursing students were active participants in these and other local and regional conferences, workshops, and symposia. A special workshop was organized in May 2006 on transcultural nursing and featured a renowned transcultural nurse leader. In April 2007 at the second International Nursing Conference, two senior nursing students presented papers. These activities have afforded students a rich opportunity to meet and network with nursing leaders from all over the world, as well as develop leadership skills for their own cultural context.

Unexpected Challenges

The primary clinical site identified for nursing students in the collaborative relationship with the Dar Al Hekma nursing program was King Faisal Specialist Hospital in Jeddah. Because the facility had only 250 beds, it became necessary to collaborate with other hospitals and health centers in the region to provide a rich and varied clinical experience for students. Some hospitals were not able to provide clinical rotations because of existing exclusive agreements with the major university in the region. An additional challenge that arose related to payment of tuition. Students who attend the local university did not pay tuition, as higher education in the kingdom is free. In addition, students at university get a monthly stipend. As a private college, it became necessary to constantly tout the "quality education" of Dar Al Hekma as a major strength and selling factor. Other hospitals were not interested in providing scholarships for students, as it was believed to be more cost effective to hire nurses from the Philippines or India rather than sponsor a Saudi baccalaureate nursing student. The worldwide shortage of nurses and the need for a stable workforce was not recognized by some hospital administrators and community leaders at the time.

A major challenge in developing agreements with international universities related to the security of the region. Negotiations with Melbourne University in Australia had been under way for some time when terrorist events occurred in Riyadh and other parts of the kingdom. The projected proposal would involve faculty/student exchange, curriculum review, and development of a master's program in nursing. Plans fell through because of insecurities of travel on behalf of both parties.

Currently the Ministry of Higher Education is resistant to programs offered solely via distance learning. It may take some time to overcome this barrier, and until then, the advantage of distance education for degree programs in Saudi Arabia is not an option.

Other challenges related to nursing preceptors appointed by the hospital with different role expectations and job titles. At one point, it became necessary to assign a staff development instructor to work full-time with Dar Al Hekma nursing students, thus decreasing instructional resources for hospital nurses.

Lessons Learned

The program is in its fifth year, and it is much too early to be able to measure its long term effect on nursing. Two students graduated in June 2006, and nine students graduated in February 2007. However, the potential impact these students can have on the advancement of nursing in Saudi Arabia is unlimited.

A major lesson learned by all parties is that a strategic partnership requires teamwork and a strong commitment to the long-term goals and objectives of the program. Excellent communication is required to ensure the trust and sharing needs for effective collaboration. Because the institutions were located in different parts of the city of Jeddah, keeping faculty and staff well informed about plans and changes involved a good deal of travel time and energy, especially with some of the travel and chaperone constraints that are unique to women in Saudi Arabia.

In spite of minor frustrations, the satisfaction that comes from being a part of a project such as this is like "polishing diamonds." Nurses are an essential asset to health care in any country, and to work with colleagues to advance the nursing profession in a country where professional nurses are a scare resource was most rewarding. In Saudi Arabia, baccalaureate nurse graduates are truly diamonds and deserving of a quality nursing education. This partnership model was a small, but important step in strengthening the journey toward excellence for nurses in Saudi Arabia.

3

SUCCESS IN PREPARATION OF FUTURE NURSE SCIENTISTS AND NURSE LEADERS: A GLOBAL PERSPECTIVE

JOYCE J. FITZPATRICK, PhD, RN, FAAN

There are several dimensions of achieving success globally, all of which depend on the structure and processes that are developed and implemented to provide a firm foundation for programmatic initiatives. Globalization of the nursing program of the Frances Payne Bolton School of Nursing (FPB) was a direct result of a strategic planning effort undertaken in the early 1990s when the school was positioning itself for the next decade. The environmental scan identified strengths in the new university administration's desire to have a global presence and the awareness that competing top schools of nursing nationally also had strong global programs. In fact, our perception was that to maintain a national position of leadership, it was imperative for FPB to move into the global arena. Thus, the journey began, and the school was immersed in global partnerships. All of the efforts were systematically developed, and while all were successful, some have been easier to sustain. Most importantly, the key ingredient of all of the partnerships has been the strong nurse leaders that provided the linkages from the other countries. Thus, this is not the story of one person, or even one school of nursing, but rather the story of leaders in nursing from many countries, all of whom joined forces and pooled resources to advance both nursing science and professional practice.

This success story details a glimpse of the leadership initiatives developed in partnership with others. While several examples are included, they are not exhaustive of the many networks that were woven together over time. Most of the partnerships continue today, and new ones have been built on the strong foundation developed through the World Health Organization (WHO) Collaborating Center for Nursing and Midwifery that exists at FPB.

GLOBAL PERSPECTIVE OF CASE WESTERN RESERVE UNIVERSITY (CASE)

If you stay long enough in a position as dean you will experience the transition of key leaders in the university administration. While I had a long, 15-and-a-half year tenure as dean of the FPB School of Nursing, so also did the presidents of CASE. In fact, there were only two presidents of CASE during my tenure, providing stability in leadership that contributed greatly to the success of the FPB global initiatives. Prior to the appointment of the new president of the university in 1990, CASE had a strong regional and national presence, but the new administration challenged the university to become committed locally and globally, describing these new dimensions as characteristics of a great university. This new perspective provided the support for FPB to extend its reach globally.

One of the initial international projects of FPB was built on another major university strength within the school of medicine. Dr. Fred Robbins, former dean of the CASE School of Medicine, former executive director of the Institute of Medicine, and a Nobel Prize winner, had developed research partnerships in Uganda. Through his efforts and the existing partnership that FPB had with the Frontier School of Midwifery in Hyden, Kentucky, we were able to successfully compete for one of two Rockefeller Foundation grants that were earmarked for US schools of nursing willing to partner in an African country.

LAUNCHING A WHO COLLABORATING CENTER

The initial application for designation as a WHO Collaborating Center for Nursing and Midwifery was planned for more than 2 years before it was officially launched. A systematic analysis was undertaken to determine how to position FPB was success. The most important criterion was to demonstrate that the initiative would not be duplicative of WHO Centers that existed in other schools of nursing in the US. FPB has received recent funding to launch a home care program, and no other schools were strategically positioned in home care nursing. The FPB Collaborating Center for Nursing and Midwifery has been successfully sustained since its inception in 1993. The roots are strong and the branches and flowers of the initial effort are many and varied. Several dozen faculty members from FPB have participated in the many programs, and partnerships now exist in Africa, Asia, Australia, Europe, and North, Central, and South America.

MAJOR PARTNERSHIPS ON THE AFRICAN CONTINENT

Uganda: *The Women for Women's Health Project.* Through major funding of the Rockefeller Foundation, FPB partnered with Makerere University Faculty of Medicine to create the first baccalaureate program in nursing (BSN) in Uganda. Six nurse faculty members were recruited to the graduate program at FPB and were prepared as core faculty for the new BSN program. While the Ugandan nurses were studying at FPB, faculty was sent to Uganda to develop and teach the beginning BSN courses. This partnership with Makerere University was later extended to focus on preparing health professional students (medicine, nursing, dentistry, and public health) to address health-care issues related to the human immunodeficiency virus (HIV/AIDS) pandemic. Dozens of CASE nursing, medical, and public health students have studied in Uganda and launched collaborative training and research projects as a result of the strong partnership that exists between the two universities.

Zimbabwe: *The MSN Distance Learning Project.* Based on the success of the Uganda project, and the FPB commitment to advancing nursing in Africa, the Kellogg Foundation provided funding for the development of the first graduate program in nursing in sub Sahara Africa. Nurse leaders were recruited from neighboring countries as well. Faculty members from FPB spent 6 weeks to 6 months in residence in Harare, Zimbabwe, throughout the 3 years of the funded project. Recently, one of the nurses who completed her master's degree as part of the initial cohort of nurses defended her PhD dissertation at CASE. She undoubtedly will continue in a leadership position locally, regionally, and globally.

MAJOR PARTNERSHIPS FOR PREPARING NURSES WITH DOCTORATES

Ireland: *Funding for two nurses selected from a national competition in Ireland was provided by two local Cleveland-based foundations interested in addressing the global shortage of nurses.* The rationale was to prepare the nurses at the highest academic level so that they might provide leadership for future development in their home countries. Nursing in Ireland has changed dramatically since that time, with all nursing education now at the university level in Ireland, a change that seemed distant when the partnership was initiated. One of the FPB alumni, Dr. Geraldine McCarthy, is now dean of the School of Nursing and Midwifery at University College Cork and is a leader in Irish nursing.

Thailand: *Through funding by the Thai government and the championship of Dr. Tasana Boontang, several nurses were supported to obtain graduate degrees at US universities.* Since launching partnerships between several Thai universities and FPB, more than 20 nurses have obtained master's and doctoral (PhD) degrees at CASE. To receive funding the individuals were expected to return to Thailand to provide leadership for research and practice development. As a result of the partnerships, several research collaborations are ongoing, and FPB graduates now populate the Thailand nursing leadership ranks.

Korea: *Partnerships built on individual leaders.* The Korean connection was initiated by one interested Korean-American faculty member at FPB, Dr. HaeOk Lee, who was committed to sharing intellectual resources with colleagues in Korea. Through her efforts a number of Korean nurses were recruited to FPB to study at the master's and doctoral level. Several collaborative research projects were initiated, including the first United Nations Development Project (UNDP) to be awarded to a nurse. This project led to the rehabilitation and deinstitutionalization of large numbers of mentally ill persons in South Korea and was recognized at the highest level in the country and through Sigma Theta Tau International (STTI) nursing honorary society. The project continues today and has been expanded in reach and influence through the tireless efforts of Dr. Susie Kim.

PARTNERSHIPS TO PROVIDE LEADERSHIP TRAINING IN HOME CARE

Several international projects have been focused on home care based on the WHO Collaborating Center concentration in this area. In 1994 a home-care conference was held in Padua and Venice, Italy, in which nurses from throughout Europe participated. As a result of this conference, a home-care book was published, featuring the collaborative efforts of several nurse leaders. In this same year home-care conferences titled "East Meets West in Home Care" were held in both Korea and Thailand. Several hundred nurses participated. In both 1995 and 1996 a

Home Care Leadership Training Program for Korean nurse leaders was held for 3 weeks each summer in Cleveland.

ADDITIONAL PARTNERSHIPS

The examples presented here are but the tip of the iceberg of partnerships developed and collaborative efforts to advance nursing globally. Partnerships exist in many other countries. As many as 200 nurses have visited FPB annually; many are interested in collaborative research or advanced educational partnerships. Many partners are from resource-rich countries, but just as many are from countries rich in people resources, but poor in monetary support. Thus, philanthropy is important, as are institutional partnerships. We have successfully obtained program support from multinational corporations interested in investing in nurses and nursing as a link to employee and public health.

SUMMARY

The benefits of the global partnerships are many. Partnerships developed early in the 1990s have now blossomed, and new projects have taken root from the beginning seeds that were planted. Alumni throughout the globe are connected to FPB based on the partnerships developed and sustained. The approach has consistently been to prepare those who could serve as country leaders in development of nursing science and professional practice so that they can influence future generations of nurses. The ripple effort is never-ending, as current student nurses in many of the countries now recount to me the influence of those that I mentored years ago. While it is possible to record the outcomes in the usual academic manner, that is, articles published and grants funded (and all of these dimensions point to major successes), the intangible rewards are noteworthy. Nursing is a built on interpersonal relationships, and it is these relationships that have made all of my global efforts successful. At a minimum, thousands of nurses' professional lives have been influenced. Thus, there has been a concomitant effect on the health of individuals, families, communities, countries, and the world in which we live. Undoubtedly, the world is a better place because of the partnerships that have been initiated, implemented, and sustained.

LESSONS LEARNED, CHALLENGES AND OPPORTUNITIES, AND ADVICE FOR FUTURE GENERATIONS OF LEADERS AND TRAVELERS

While my goal in life has always been to "hold an endowed chair on Pan Am," international work is not for the easily fatigued. International work is *hard work.* Flexibility in all endeavors is a key to success. Whether you are participating in a meeting held in the King of Jordan's conference room, hosted by one of his ministers, or sitting on the ground collecting data with grandmothers in the villages of Uganda, the energy level required is high. Another important factor to consider is that when you are in another country, you are a guest of those who live there. Their customs, their rituals, and their patterns should be honored, and you should always defer to their choices of activities and schedules. Another element of global partnership is the resource requirement that is necessary to launch and sustain quality programs. Global work is resource intensive, particularly as nothing replaces the face-to-face contact on which many partnerships are based. International work is about relationships between and among individuals; thus, it is most important to connect and sustain the personal contact. Of course, now the connections are facilitated by the ease of electronic communication and the frequency of international conferences.

Importantly, international connections require a long-term investment. Relationships are not spontaneously developed, nor are collaborative projects. Investments must be mutual, although they do not have to be equal or the same. The time and energy of individuals are crucial components for sustaining the momentum and solidifying the projects and programs. The future holds so many opportunities, and I thoroughly enjoy being the connector. If I am talking with a nurse in Boston who has an idea for a project that I know is of interest in Beijing, I marvel at the enthusiasm of the potential partners and the ease of connection. For me, the rewards are in the professional relationships developed to advance nursing. While, of course, some always see insurmountable challenges, I am constantly reminded of my favorite leadership incentive:

"Nothing will ever be attempted if all possible objections must first be overcome"
—Samuel Johnson

4

THE INTERNATIONAL NETWORK FOR DOCTORAL EDUCATION IN NURSING: A SUCCESS STORY

SHAKÉ KETEFIAN, EDD, RN, FAAN

A rapid increase in nursing doctoral education worldwide was becoming manifest in the mid- to late 1990s; the growth in nursing science was a reflection of this program growth and the concomitant increase in graduates holding nursing doctorates. With these developments, educators felt a need to create a mechanism to network together and discuss issues of mutual interest. This is the story of the creation and subsequent development of the International Network for Doctoral Education in Nursing (INDEN), from its inception to the present.

THE BEGINNINGS

The beginnings of INDEN can be traced to a national meeting of the annual forum for doctoral education in the United States (US), held at the University of Michigan (UM) in 1995. This forum had begun in the 1970s to enable doctoral educators and deans to convene each year to discuss issues related to doctoral education, research, and the development of nursing science. Traditionally, schools rotated hosting responsibilities for these meetings. The 1995 meeting was the annual meeting of the doctoral forum hosted by the UM. For the first time in the history of the doctoral forum, the organizers had invited several international speakers and representatives of international doctoral programs—several of whom participated—to attend.

During this 2-day meeting the group avidly discussed the idea of forming a parallel international doctoral forum similar to the US group; this was deemed necessary and quite valuable to international doctoral educators. While most attendees supported the initiative, concern evolved over the possible undermining of activities that could occur with two such groups, US and international, in existence. Discussion revealed that the informal doctoral forum may have met its goals, because nursing doctoral programs had expanded dramatically and nursing research was well established and maturing. Thus, the doctoral forum decided to commission a survey of its members as to the continuing need for the forum and to obtain the members' views on dissolving the US forum and, in its place, establishing an international group concerned with doctoral education globally.

The study was conducted, and a report was presented to the doctoral forum membership the following year. The main finding and recommendation was to dissolve the forum and establish an international group; the report further recommended that an international meeting on doctoral education be organized before the International Council of Nurses (ICN) Congress in 1997 in Vancouver, Canada. Such a meeting was organized and held on the campus of the University of British Columbia (UBC). This choice of venue enabled the conference registration to be affordable, and the meeting succeeded in attracting a large international contingent of doctoral educators. One hundred professionals attended the one-day meeting, and interest in the creation of an international organization remained high. By convening informal biennial meetings before or following other international meetings, we were able to attract a broader audience of constituents. Thus, the next meeting was held in London in 1999, preceding the centennial conference of ICN. At this time, the decision was made to formalize the group and to begin developing bylaws to govern the group's operation and activities. Subsequently, drafts were prepared and circulated and then were approved at the next meeting held before ICN in Copenhagen in 2001. Officers and board members were elected via electronic communication. With officers in place, the new organization was off to a good start and was housed at the UM.

INDEN was created because participants in the meetings felt a need to have such a group where collegial dialogue could take place and where informal advice could be sought and ideas tried in a safe environment. Thus, the overall aim of INDEN, as declared on their web site, is to advance and promote high quality doctoral education in nursing through national/international collaboration" (INDEN, n.d.). Thus, interest on the development of standards to improve the quality of doctoral programs worldwide became a first priority. A task force was convened, with representatives of nine countries charged with developing quality criteria, standards, and indicators. The group was to work for 4 years before a report could be submitted to the board and the membership for discussion and approval. This was clearly a milestone. By then INDEN had a web site, and the document on doctoral program quality was the first major report to be displayed. The sheer process of moving such an international task force (and subsequent committees) was an important learning accomplishment for all involved. With diverse models and types of doctoral education worldwide and different foci, the learning process began. The criteria, standards, and indicators to be developed had to be responsive to various models of doctoral education, although the group established some parameters, without which the task would have been nearly impossible. The decision was made to focus only on doctoral programs that aimed to develop research expertise in students. Therefore, the document was applicable to research-focused doctoral programs, regardless of the modes of instruction; this meant that the document would apply to doctoral education where no coursework was required and where research occurred under the supervision of one faculty member, as is the case in most of Europe. It would also apply to programs with formal coursework combined with independent study and dissertation with supervision by a team of faculty members, as is the case in North America.

Several additional initiatives were established at the outset to assist the organization in setting a course for itself. Committees were formed to address recommendations for doctoral/postdoctoral workshops; a plan for research interest groups to promote international research collaboration; a commission to make recommendations for ways in which institutions can collaborate in facilitating student and faculty exchange opportunities to enrich learning; a task force to develop worldwide research priorities for nurse scholars in an effort to make their research more responsive to societal needs; and a task force to develop guidance for mentorship that would be applicable worldwide. In addition to these initiatives, the Board of Directors (BoD) and committee chairs engaged in a strategic planning process. As a result of these initiatives, the organization is focused on the following activities:

1. **Doctoral/postdoctoral workshops**: Using our members in different regions of the world, INDEN collaborates with them and their institutions to develop and offer workshops for doctoral students and those in early stages of their postdoctoral careers. These events are usually connected to large international conferences, occurring immediately before or immediately after such conferences without interfering with those conference schedules.

2. **Postdoctoral fellowships**: INDEN and Sigma Theta Tau International (STTI) are collaborating to jointly offer a 3-month postdoctoral mentoring fellowship. These competitive fellowships are need-based. The goal is to mentor them in their own research and at the same time to help them become effective mentors of their own doctoral students. Selection occurs by an international committee. Once selected, the fellows are placed in institutions that offer research-intensive environments where an

experienced faculty member with similar research interests provides supervision to the fellow.

3. **Biennial scientific conferences**: The membership of INDEN meets every 2 years for a scientific meeting as well as to conduct the business of the organization. Each scientific meeting has a theme, and leaders from various parts of the world are invited as speakers. Throughout the 2 days, time is allocated to conduct the business of INDEN, to update members on activities of the previous biennium, and to develop plans for the next biennium to guide the BoD in its work, because the board is responsible for the conduct of the organization's work between meetings.

4. **Publications**: To communicate with members on a regular basis and to provide a forum for dialogue, a newsletter was created, which is published three times a year, circulated to members, and placed on the web site.

A major publication initiative was the publication of a book on international doctoral education, edited by two of the co-founders of INDEN (Ketefian & McKenna, 2005). Thirty individuals, many of whom are INDEN members with expertise in different areas of doctoral education, contributed chapters. All chapters were written by teams of two or more authors from different countries. This ensured that a variety of perspectives are represented in the discussion of the issue at hand

During the planning of the book it was agreed that all royalties generated from the sale of the book would be donated to INDEN, to be used for INDEN's programming for students and postdoctoral scholars. Each contributor author also agreed to forego the payment from the publisher toward the same end.

IMPACT AND DEVELOPMENTS TO DATE

INDEN is an individual membership organization. In many respects it is an online academic community in that the majority of its work is conducted electronically, through e-mail and its web site. The founders and all participating members expressed a commitment in the early meetings that membership dues would be designed in such a way that any eligible faculty member or doctoral student from anywhere would not be precluded from joining because of high dues. This was taken to heart by the first board. Thus, a three-tier dues structure was developed following the general approach used by the ICN, using country income/development levels from the World Bank data. Three "bands" were thus created and dues were set accordingly; in addition, for doctoral students a separate, lower level of dues was established, thus creating three levels of dues, with regular and student dues for each level, for a total of six different categories of dues.

This complicated system was presented in a simplified manner on a membership page on the web site, using a secure system provided by the UM. Individuals can sign up and pay dues online. We maintain a mailing list of doctoral programs, with 355 international doctoral programs offered in 34 countries. We have 238 active members representing 24 of the 34 countries offering nursing doctoral education; one third of the members are doctoral students.

INDEN's central tenet has been collaborative and consultative. Such collaboration pervades all aspects of the work, whether it is in the work of the board or officers or in the manner in which the committees function. Collaboration is the key to success producing documented results. We consider multiple perspectives to ensure relevance to members from all countries. When we form committees or conduct elections, the composition of the groups has to generally reflect the composition of the overall membership. For example, the current board represents seven countries; additionally, given the number of student members, two members of the board are elected students with full privileges, although they are not asked to chair committees unless they wish to be so involved and feel ready to undertake leadership roles within the organization.

MEASURES OF SUCCESS

By any measure, INDEN has been a success, and its impact is being felt in many parts of the world. What then accounts for this? Several factors can be identified and are described here:

1. **Inclusiveness.** Early board decisions regarding membership dues structure and continuing efforts to reach out to doctoral educators and students everywhere to embrace them within the organization found resonance with the members. Similarly, elections are conducted with a view to developing a slate with as wide a representation as possible, resulting in a board that has had members from five to eight countries at any given time.

2. **Doctoral students.** As an important constituency of INDEN composing one-third of the membership, doctoral students hold two slots on the elected BoD. This feature ensures that organizational decisions are made in a way that is sensitive to students' situations and their professional needs. An important consideration in INDEN programming is to develop activities that will meet their needs. Examples are student seminars organized in various regions, efforts to organize biennial meetings in ways that will enable them to network together, and the like. At the recommendation of students we have instituted a display of student posters at biennial meetings. This provides students an opportunity to obtain early experience in preparing scholarly presentations with their advisors' guidance. They meet scholars during the biennial meetings and explain their work. It also makes it possible for students to seek funding to attend the INDEN meetings. The organization allocates funds in its conference budgets to provide partial travel subsidies to students from middle- and low-income countries who are presenting their posters. We also invite students to glean leadership skills by participating on task forces and committees as members, enabling them to learn from experienced educators how such activities are carried out.

3. **Responsiveness to member needs.** The viability of an organization depends on its ability to meet and respond to member needs. In the case of INDEN this has been and continues to be a challenge. This is especially so given that doctoral education worldwide varies greatly, from programs that are highly advanced and mature, with highly experienced educators/investigators residing in resource-rich countries, on the one hand to programs that are new and struggling, where junior faculty are asked to function as senior educators and where access to resources is a daily challenge, on the other. The needs of these groups are vastly different. However, tuning in on faculty dialogues around discussion tables at INDEN meetings and in informal dialogues reveals that they share many common interests and concerns, and members derive great satisfaction from this type of interchange and the opportunities it affords to be helpful and supportive of one another.

4. **Research needs.** Research needs of many countries are great, with limited numbers of qualified individuals to engage in research. Cognizant of this reality, INDEN encourages cross-national research involving teams and promotes the idea of doctoral

students and scholars from anywhere conducting research on problems of developing countries. Teaming up with colleagues from resource-poor countries to study compelling health problems produces knowledge that can improve health, making research more immediately applicable, and enables novice scholars from host countries to gain experience in research while contributing their knowledge of the local health problems, the customs, and the culture to make the resulting research more culturally appropriate and relevant. Toward this end, an INDEN committee developed research priorities for different regions of the world so that all individuals would be able to see the areas of regional research priorities and needs. The document on research priorities was compiled through a strategy that combined approaches involving literature searches, formal statements of professional societies, member input, interviews with leaders in various countries, and the like.

INDEN has evolved over the past 7 years to advance and promote high quality doctoral nursing education through national and international collaboration. Although our numbers are small, our goals are high. We have major accomplishments and will continue to grow.

REFERENCES

INDEN. (n.d.). Aims and Procedures of INDEN. Retreived 27 September 2007 from http://www.umich.edu/~inden/about/aims.html.

Ketefian, S., & McKenna, H. P. (Eds.) (2005). *Doctoral education in nursing: International perspectives*. London: Routledge.

5

A Global Nursing Experience: Serving Vulnerable Communities

Maureen Kelley, CNM, PhD, FACNM
Marla E. Salmon, ScD, RN, FAAN

The Nell Hodgson Woodruff School of Nursing (NHWSN) at Emory University has carefully developed its mission and vision to reflect its global context. Indeed, we are physically located between the Rollins School of Public Health and the Centers for Disease Control and Prevention (CDC) and within a city that houses The Carter Center, MedShare, and CARE. The school has defined its values as those of scholarship, leadership, and social responsibility. It is further committed to nurturing an organizational culture in which all of its members are dedicated to improving the health of vulnerable people worldwide. The school's Lillian Carter Center for International Nursing (LLCIN) was dedicated by President Carter in 1991 specifically to enable nursing to address health needs worldwide. The center and the school operate within a framework of partnership and respect for the global environment in which we function.

The school's commitment to global well-being reflects the broader university's vision, which includes working collaboratively for positive transformation in the world through "courageous leadership in teaching, research, scholarship, health care, and social action" (Emory University School of Nursing, n.d.). This vision is reflected in a strategic plan that encompasses a focus on internationalization and creating community-engaged scholars. The school's own strategic plan is closely aligned with that of the university. The purpose of this chapter is to describe a unique service-learning partnership program that has profoundly enriched the educational and cultural environment of the school and it faculty, staff, and students. This project is firmly rooted in the context of the school, university, and overall community.

DESCRIPTION OF PROJECT

The project was made possible with the generous support of the O.C. Hubert Charitable Trust. The vision and energy of faculty, staff, and students were aimed at focusing on improved health services for vulnerable populations around the world. The trust has had a strong interest in the convergence of religion, spirituality, and health. Because faith-based organizations play crucial roles in meeting health needs in the world's poorest countries, the school sees the Hubert Trust as an important partner. The school was funded to launch the Hubert International Nursing Fellows Program. The Hubert fellows, along with faculty advisers, would participate in service learning programs that include working with international faith-based organizations in developing countries. The fellowship would be implemented through an innovative Alternative Spring Break Program experience, initially funded by the O.C. Hubert Charitable Trust. The project would be coordinated through the Office of Service Learning, the unit responsible for leadership, coordination, and support of domestic and international service learning experiences for students, in partnership with the faculty and administration.

IDENTIFICATION OF FAITH-BASED ORGANIZATION PARTNER

Our first goal was to identify a partner that was well-established and respected in a community of need. The LCCIN has a strong partnership with the Caribbean Government Chief Nursing Officers through its work with the Regional Nursing Body of the Caribbean Community (CARICOM). Collaborating with these government nursing leaders and networking with faith communities resulted in our contacting the Missionaries of the Poor (MOP) in inner-city Kingston, Jamaica. This organization was brought to our attention through a request from an Atlanta nursing leader who was partnering with Emory in exploring magnet hospital status with our Caribbean partners. She became aware of a need/request from MOP for a kidney transplant for one of their brothers with end-stage renal disease. A partnership among several Atlanta hospitals resulted in a successful transplant, and the partnership was launched.

MOP is an international Catholic monastic order of brothers dedicated to serving the poorest of the poor. In Jamaica, they house and provide total care to more than 450 homeless, including physically and mentally handicapped persons and those living with HIV/AIDS. They welcome volunteers, and at the time that we contacted them, were very interested in partnering with nurses. The brothers do not have formal health training and were interested in developing a curriculum that would give them some basic knowledge and guidance on the health issues facing their residents. One of the long-term US volunteers was a nurse, and she was eager to collaborate with a school of nursing. A lead faculty made a site visit to Jamaica, meeting with the MOP and with Thelma Campbell, Chief Nursing Officer of Jamaica. Father HoLung, the founder of the community, stressed their mission as being "care not cure." He shared that many times health professional volunteers came to their centers with a first-world view of how things should be changed in the centers. They did not at first understand the power of touch, of love, of simple caring for these residents in an atmosphere of joyful service to the poor. We agreed that this would be a priority in our work with the brothers. Work the first year would include supporting the residents in activities of daily living, wound care, hospice care, and, for the faculty, a needs assessment of the type of education program that would be helpful to new brothers.

DEVELOPMENT OF ALTERNATE SPRING BREAK PROGRAM

Faculty worked with the Office of Service Learning and the LCCIN to develop the Alternate Spring Break Program. Students submit an application that addresses their interest in international service learning and how this interest fits with career and life goals. Faculty members evaluate the applications and selects the fellows. Expectations for participation in the program include the following:

- Attendance at a series of four seminars that prepare students and faculty for their settings. This includes an orientation to the faith-based organization and setting; an orientation to the host country including cultural, economic, and health considerations; a discussion of international travel and safety; and a discussion about spirituality and health/faith and health.

- Work 8–10 hours a day in the centers, participation in spiritual life of the community, discussions with nursing leaders of Jamaica, and a tour of one of the public hospitals

- Daily debriefing regarding the experiences in the centers, which serve as a forum for students and faculty to share a wide range of emotional, spiritual, sociopolitical, and cultural observations that result from their day.

- Daily journaling regarding personal reflections on the meaning and experience of the trip. This serves as an alternative way of giving voice to the experience.

- Post-trip reunion/debriefing serves to give faculty and students the opportunity to share their re-entry experience and reflect on the meaning of the trip. It also serves as another support mechanism for group members.

- Evaluation of the program. Trip members are asked to provide a structured written evaluation of the experience from the orientation session to the post-trip debriefing. This gives us feedback to better plan for future programs.

PROGRAM IMPLEMENTATION

The fellowship has just completed its third year with this faith-based organization. Students uniformly see it as a life-changing experience. They see brothers providing daily loving care to profoundly handicapped people. They see residents who form a community of support for each other. Representative comments include "This has been one of the most powerful experiences of my life, and I will carry this experience with me as I pursue a career in nursing," "The MOP is about caring for people. It is in these moments of care-holding someone's hand, offering water, that we truly make a difference," and "This week has given me a new perspective on faith and nursing, a perspective that will cause me to look deeper into the heart and soul of patients to try to find their faith/health connection. I have always considered myself a nurse that provides holistic care, but I can honestly say I have now lived and experienced holistic nursing."

UNEXPECTED CHALLENGES AND OPPORTUNITIES

One challenge we face are the inherent dangers in places that have the greatest need. For example, the U.S Department of State describes Kingston, Jamaica, as a place where gang violence and shootings occur regularly in certain areas, along with increased prevalence of violent crime (US Department of State, 2006). Two years ago, two of the brothers were murdered at the MOP monastery in an apparent random shooting. In addition, because of a recent malaria outbreak in Kingston, travelers to the area are advised to have malaria prophylaxis. We have to be able to balance working in an inner city international environment that is classified as "dangerous" with the opportunity to safely expose our students to an amazing connection and opportunity for personal and professional growth. We have been developing expertise in the administrative aspects of these international connections, including nursing licensure in the host country, memoranda of understanding, code of conduct for students, safety planning/emergency evacuation, and informed consent. We are committed to supporting the roles of leadership in nursing in the countries in which we have educational/service learning opportunities. Therefore, we make a real effort to connect our students with nursing leadership and ensure that we are following regulations for practice in the host country. We also place a special emphasis on cultural preparation of the students so that they have a beginning understanding of the context in which they will be working.

Also, a huge opportunity for flexibility offered itself to us on a daily basis. Each day, we would need to respond to multiple unanticipated requests or changes in schedule. I consider it one of the real growth opportunities that we all had—students and faculty alike.

It takes a tremendous amount of commitment to sustain these partnerships. In addition to providing volunteer services, we are committed to trying to help facilitate system improvements in ways that are strategic and meaningful to the partner organization. For example, it has been challenging to develop the "health curriculum" while we are onsite supporting the students. It is likewise challenging for the brothers to balance their need for sustained spiritual development with their interest in being better able to meet the health needs of the residents through a health curriculum and orientation program for the new brothers. In some ways it is a question of competing priorities; in others it is a matter of trusting that things are moving forward in the best way possible given everyone's best intentions.

Another long-term challenge has been to consider how to enhance the connection between this faith-based organization, which receives no government funding except antiretroviral therapy for its human immunodeficiency virus (HIV)–positive residents, with appropriate government partners. As described in a recent WHO report, there needs to be greater dialogue and action between religious and public health leaders. Specific areas of focus for this dialogue include development of religious and public health literacy, along with respectful engagement that can serve to bring together these leaders to encourage long-term collaboration in policy-making and project implementation (WHO, 2007). Again, this is a long-range goal that we would feel privileged to help facilitate.

LESSONS LEARNED

- Funding is a challenge. We are continuing to search for a stable source of funding for these types of international experiences.

- A real need for preparation exists, both cultural and emotional. That is why we use the service-learning model and require that students complete a pre-trip curriculum that includes conversations with previous trip participants. In addition, when at the international site, students journal and debrief daily with the faculty leaders. This provides a wonderful opportunity for sharing and support. We prepare students for "re-entry" and the need to re-acclimate to a first-world environment after their immersion in another culture. We also have a reunion following the trip, which serves to support the students and faculty and cement the lessons learned and directions for the future.

WORDS OF WISDOM

- If you cannot foresee sticking it out for the long haul, do not commit.

- Partnerships go both directions.

- There is a need for a feedback loop and a primary "point person" for the project.

- It is worth it to implement these kinds of experiences for students and faculty. It is a wonderful privilege to be a witness to the way that this experience touches the hearts and minds of our students.

- The school has to live its values across the enterprise.

- The school needs to have and expect partnership between staff and faculty.

REFERENCES

Emory University School of Nursing. (n.d.). Mission, Vision, and Values. Retrieved 27 September 2007 from http://www.nursing.emory.edu/nursing/about/mission.shtml.

US Department of State. (December 20, 2006). Consular information sheet: Jamaica. *Travel. state.gov: Bureau of Consular Affairs*. Retrieved 27 September 2007 from http://travel.state. gov/travel/cis_pa_tw/cis/cis_1147.html.

World Health Organization. (8 February 2007). Faith-based organizations play a major role in HIV/AIDS care and treatment in Sub-Saharan Africa. *Note for the Press*. Retrieved 27 September 2007 from http://www.who.int/hiv/mediacentre/news66/en/index.html.

6

International Collaborative Initiatives for Nurses

Mary Paterson, PhD, RN
Patricia C. McMullen, PhD, JD, CNS, CRNP, FNAP

Nursing is a global profession, and numerous opportunities exist for nurses to work together to advance the profession. Several federal programs exist that provide excellent opportunities for nurses to dialogue, with the ultimate goal of not only enhancing the profession, but also improving health care for literally thousands of people. Here, we share two stories of successful international partnerships that benefited both nurses in the United States (US) and those from distant nations.

The Kosovo–Catholic University of America Experience

The Hope Fellowship Program (HF) represents a unique partnership between the United States Agency for International Development (USAID) and the Balkan countries—Albania, Kosovo, Macedonia, and Montenegro. According to their web site, the purpose of the program is to "facilitate vision, multi-ethnic leadership development with women and men throughout the Balkans" (Hope Fellowship Program, n.d.). HF empowers these leaders to create collaborative, sustainable, positive change in government, civil society, and business that strengthens the democratic process and promotes prosperity for all people in the region.

Historically, nursing education in Kosovo has been rooted in secondary schools, with students completing 8 years of basic education and 4 years of nursing education at the high-school level. Nurses and midwives provide more than 50% of all health-care services in the country, but salaries, autonomy, and status within the health professions are low (Huruglica, 2004). In 2004 no national nursing licensure existed, nor were standardized core nursing competencies established via nursing school curricula or a licensure examination.

As a consequence of widespread shifts in both governmental policies and in health care, Fetije (Feta) Huruglica, Chief Nursing Officer (CNO) of the Kosovo Ministry of Health (MOH), was sponsored by the Hope Fellowship Program to explore nursing licensure and educational issues with nurses and health policy experts in the US. Feta received her nursing education at the Pristina Secondary Medical School and has worked for over 27 years in hospitals, community-based clinics, and mobile clinics. From March to June of 1999, she had provided critical nursing care to displaced Kosovar citizens in the Macedonia Border Region. Under a newly developing government and health-care system, Feta was appointed as the Chief of the Nursing Division of the Kosovo MOH and serves as the voice for more than 7,000 nurses employed by the Kosovo Health System.

A tremendous benefit of the Hope Fellowship Program is the support courses that they offer. Fellows receive valuable didactic content and practice experiences in the areas of leadership, advocacy, and public speech. Additionally, they have a detailed orientation concerning American cultural norms and valuable training on working within the US.

Before coming to the US, Feta and Drs. Ann Marie Brooks and Patricia McMullen used e-mail to establish learning competencies for Feta's experience. The four main competencies that were negotiated were as follows: (1) analyze the process of nursing licensure in the US, with emphasis on both the process and current issues concerning licensure; (2) describe approaches to baccalaureate nursing education in the US; (3) analyze the development of health care and nursing in the US; and (4) assess future health-care initiatives in the US. Dialogue opportunities all focused on these four competencies.

To gain information on nursing licensure in the US, Feta had extended meetings with the Maryland and District of Columbia boards of nursing. Over the course of these experiences, she was able to gain insight on the differences between licensure and certification, levels of licensure, core nursing curricula, and the Interstate Nurse Licensure Compact (https://www.ncsbn.org/156.htm). Licensure experts also provided her with web site locations that were helpful when she returned to Kosovo. Nursing education competencies were addressed via experiences conducted at the offices of the American Association of Colleges of Nursing (AACN) and through collaborative experiences with nurses at both the Catholic University of America (CUA) and neighboring schools of nursing. Policy issues that affect and shape the roles of nurses in America were explored by discussion and review of such health-care initiatives as Healthy People 2010: Agenda for Health Care in America (Healthy People 2010, 2000) and Put Prevention into Practice (Agency for Healthcare Research and Quality, 1998).

Since her Hope Fellowship, Feta and nurse colleagues from Kosovo and other countries have made groundbreaking advances in professional nursing. Under European Union funding, a nursing and midwifery department was founded at the University of Pristina. Standardized nursing curricula were developed for these two programs, and following 3 years of intensive study, graduates are awarded a bachelor's degree. On 31 October 2006, 29 nurses and 18 nurse midwives became the first nurses to complete their nursing education at the collegiate level. Importantly, 47 of these nurses have been selected to pursue master's degree studies at Glasgow Caledonian University. Feta and her colleagues have also established regular international nursing conferences in Kosovo that continue to promote professional nursing within the country. More information on this international initiative is available online at http://www.kosovonursingconference.org/.

Changing Nursing's Role: Egyptian Health care Reform

Sound basic nursing education is an important first step toward the improvement of health care; another important aspect of international nursing is shaping the workplace environment to make maximum use of the skills and abilities of newly trained and retrained nurses. Primary health-care reform has been a target initiative of many international agencies including the US Agency for International Development (USAID), the World Bank, and the European Union (EU). Nursing is an important component in most of these reform programs, because nurses have traditionally been providers of much of the primary care in many nations. Primary health-care reform usually requires significant adjustments in payment systems, renovation and re-equipping of ambulatory facilities, and attention to clinical practice guidelines and pathways to promote less specialist care and more family medicine.

The primary health-care reform program in Egypt, sponsored by USAID, the World Bank, and the EU, provides an interesting example of the interaction between these systemic changes and the retraining of nurses to work as key members of the health-care team. In Egypt, a pilot program was started in Alexandria with the assistance of Dr. Mary Paterson, a US prepared registered nurse, to test the effectiveness of the new primary health-care model. As part of the pilot program, nurses and physicians were trained together for 6 months in family care teams at several training sites in the United Kingdom (UK) and US. This training emphasized a collaborative model of primary care that used the skills of the nurse to provide family-focused assessment and supportive care, as well as health education to individuals and the design and implementation of community health promotion programs. The primary health-care teams were judged a highly successful component of the Alexandria pilot program, and the collaborative model of care has been replicated in many other parts of Egypt.

It is important to note that improving the basic educational experience and licensure of nurses is an essential step toward the implementation of such health-care reform programs. Programs such as those described in Kosovo work to provide improved basic education of nurses. As the Egyptian project demonstrated, it is also important to enrich the working environment so that nurses can use their enhanced skills to the fullest extent possible to improve the health of the population. The key point is the interdependence of basic education and health system reform. One cannot be achieved without attention to the other.

REFERENCES

Agency for Healthcare Research and Quality. (1998). *Clinician's handbook of preventive services: Put prevention into practice.* (Second edition). Retrieved 27 September 2007 from http://www.ahrq.gov/clinic/ppiphand.htm.

Hope Fellowship Program. (n.d.). WLP info sheet. Retrieved 27 September 2007 from http://www.naac-hf.org/index.php?option-com_frontpage&Itemid-43.

Huruglica, F. (2004). Hope Fellowship Program Leadership Initiative. Analysis of the processes of licensure and nursing education in the United States. Washington, DC: United States Agency for International Development.

Sadiq, A., Sadiq, L., El Beih, W., Paterson, M. (2001). Evaluation of the Demonstration Project for the financing of Primary Health Care in Egypt. Washington, D.C: Abt Associates for the United States Agency for International Development.

US Department of Health and Human Services. (2000). *Healthy People 2010.* Author. Washington, D.C.

7

THE US-RUSSIAN NURSING CONFERENCE CRUISE: A CATALYST FOR COLLABORATIVE PROFESSIONAL DEVELOPMENT

MARIE J. DRIEVER, PhD, RN
RACHEL DiFAZIO, RN, MS, CPNP

Every other year since 1997, a unique nursing conference takes place on a riverboat, cruising Russia's waterways between St. Petersburg and Moscow. This biennial United States (US)-Russian Nursing Conference Cruise is unique in having Russian and US nurses participate equally as conference speakers, poster presenters, discussion group leaders, and facilitators of clinical and educational site visits.

In addition, Russian nurses share in the sightseeing, helping those from the US and other countries see and experience Russia firsthand. American nurses find conference sessions, sightseeing, meals, and other times for informal discussion provide opportunities to network and develop relationships with their Russian colleagues. The goals of the US-Russian Nursing Conference Cruise are to:

- Learn about and experience Russian culture and perspectives on nursing and healthcare delivery.

- Build collegial relationships and friendships between US and Russian nurses.

- Foster intercultural professional understanding.

- Create the basis for post-conference exchanges and collaboration.

The goal of generating post-conference exchanges and collaboration has been realized in multiple ways. Within the context of this success story, we describe the kinds of collaboration that have resulted from the Conference Cruise. These unique partnerships have promoted the professional development of US and Russian participants.

US-Russian Nursing Conference Cruise as Context for Collaboration

The US-Russian Nursing Conference developed in response to requests from Russian nurses to have more time to obtain information and interact with US colleagues during exchange visits. Russian nurses were interested in attending conferences with US colleagues that lasted longer than 3–4 days to allow for further dialog on related topics. Offering a conference on a cruise of the Russian waterways provides many benefits. The longer time afforded by a cruise, combined with the venue of being together on a boat, creates opportunities to explore topics in more depth, to have time to ask more probing questions, and to reflect on the information exchanged. It also allows time for interactions that lead to the development of collaborative relationships. This conference draws nurses, primarily from the US, but from other nations as well, and has a mission beyond leisure: to establish networks that promote scholarly international exchange and to help nursing in Russia evolve into a modern profession.

Project Description

Over the 10 years of offering the US-Russian Nursing Conference Cruise, an evolution has occurred in the kinds and numbers of professional exchanges. Initially, the focus was on US nurses developing exchanges with Russian colleagues in the form of internships and other educational activities. With the *4th US-Russian Nursing Conference Cruise* in 2003, the conference coordinators initiated another type of collaborative effort. The Conference Cruise began offering Russian participants an opportunity to submit a proposal to conduct a project after the Conference Cruise to strengthen nursing and/or health-care delivery within their respective work settings. Assisting the Russian participants in designing and implementing a project after the Conference Cruise requires collaborative support from US colleagues on a number of levels. While financial support is integral to the process, the dialogue and relationships developed during the Conference Cruise set the stage for the identification of possible projects, the organization of these ideas into a proposal, and then delineating needed resources. To identify needed resources required developing a budget as well as clarifying the in-kind resources and materials to be shared with Russian colleagues to ensure successful project completion.

Early in the 16-day Conference Cruise, the coordinators explain the project grants program and invite the Russian nurses to develop a proposal to improve nursing and/or patient care in their work settings. Discussions during the Conference Cruise provide an impetus for the development of a project proposal that is submitted at the end of the Conference Cruise by the Russian nurses. The Conference Cruise coordinators work with and mobilize US nurses to access funding resources. They seek and work with potential individuals, groups, and organizations who are likely to be interested in supporting these projects. A diverse set of sources provides the funds for the small grant awards, currently in the amount of $500 US.

DESCRIPTION OF RUSSIAN PROJECTS

Examples of Russian projects completed include:

- Development of a web site for the national nursing association of RussiaN Nursing Association (RNA).

- Integration of the use of visual aids for diabetic teaching.

- Development of pressure relieving surfaces and teaching materials for patient/families and nurses on ways to prevent nosocomial pressure ulcers.

- Development of informational brochures about the availability of hospice services.

- Development of informational brochure about surgical interventions for children with heart defects.

Please refer to Tables E-7.1 and E-7.2 for specific descriptions of the projects completed, in 2003 and 2005. In addition to financial support, US participants furthered collaborative efforts through the sharing of critical resources. US participants have aided Russian colleagues by providing teaching materials to be adapted to the Russian context. Upon completion, Russian nurses submit reports on their project achievements.

TABLE E-7.1. DESCRIPTIONS OF TWO POST-CRUISE PROJECTS.

Grant Recipient	Goal	Support
US-Russian Global Links Project	Develop a web site for the RNA; Olga Komissarova worked with two faculty from Indiana	Small grant awarded plus in-kind and monetary support from US partners
	University/Purdue in Fort Wayne, Indiana;	Six STTI chapters and others Carol Sternberger and Linda Meyer represented US
Education about Community Hospice Services	Marina Basenko of Novgorod Regional Women's Community Organization and League of Middle-Aged and Elderly Women	Funding from Dobra, Inc., a non-profit in Portland, Oregon

TABLE E-7.2. PROJECT DESCRIPTIONS: NINE RUSSIAN NURSES FOLLOWING THE 2005 CONFERENCE

Project	Goal	Support
Yuri Bessonov, Independent Researcher, Russian Nursing History, Vyborg	Pilot for social rehabilitation of spinal-cord patients through use of Internet connection to resources including support groups, create network of disabled Russians through distance education.	STTI Chapter Nu Iota, Reno, Nevada
Marina Boykova, Children's Hospital #1, St. Petersburg	Pretest research instrument, explore qualitative interview techniques, learn thematic analysis	University of Oklahoma College of Nursing
Olga Egorova, Leningrad Regional Clinical Hospital, St. Petersburg	Decrease incidence of pressure ulcers (PUs) in regional medical center	Cheryl Rowder, with in-kind support from Providence Portland Medical Center
Svetlana Korotkova, Leningrad Regional Clinical Hospital, St. Petersburg	Improve patient education for older diabetics with diabetic school model using TV, VCR, and more	Individual donor in collaboration with Dobra, Inc; resources from Sharon Ostwald, Texas

TABLE E-7.2.   PROJECT DESCRIPTIONS: 9 RUSSIAN NURSES FOLLOWING THE 2005 CONFERENCE (CONTINUED)

Project	Goal	Support
Olga Morozova, Yaroslav Community Hospice	Develop informational postcards about hospice using children's artwork to increase awareness of cancer patient's end-of-life needs and increase donations	Dobra, Inc.
Irina Ostrovskaya, Sergiev Posad Medical School and Raisa Grosheva, Health Care Administrative Department of Arkhangelsk Region	Initiate task force of RNA members to define nursing consistent with current and desired development of the profession	University of Illinois at Chicago College of Nursing
Alexandra Stupak, Suraz Central Hospital, Suraz	Create a more normal and less stressful environment for hospitalized children with TV and DVD resources	Larry Plant, director of behavioral service at Southern Maine Medical Center, Biffeford, Maine
Natalia Tsvetkova, Bakulev's State Scientific Center of Cardiovascular Surgery, Moscow	Improve parental education about availability of children's cardiac services for congenital heart disease	STTI—Beta Delta Chapter; Rachel DeFazio, Children's Hospital, Boston, Massachusetts, offered teaching resources

PROJECT SPONSORS/RESOURCE MATERIAL CONTRIBUTORS

The sources of funding and contribution of resource materials also reflect diverse interests and commitments as project funding and other support has come from:

- Individual donations

- Schools of nursing

- Individuals and a nonprofit organization

OUTCOMES ACHIEVED

In the process of completing their projects, Russian nurses are able to make a difference for patients and families as well as other nurses. These projects also provide a way for participants from the US to support their Russian colleagues and learn about project outcomes and their benefits. Through ongoing dialogue with their peers, US and Russian nurses learn about patient concerns in each other's countries and ways in which care outcomes can be improved. From anecdotal reports provided by the 10 Russian nurses who completed projects after the 2003 and 2005 Conference Cruises, we know that the grants program has contributed to improved levels of care and personal and professional growth.

Another success marker involved examining where the projects were implemented and the kinds of patient populations that were targeted. Russians nurses have completed projects in major cities of St Petersburg and Moscow and small towns such as Novgorod, Sergiev Possad, Yaroslavl, and Syrazh in the south, and Archangelsk in the far north of Russia. Thus, regardless of the oblast (province) in which one lives, success is an outcome. In addition, Russian patient populations served by these projects include parents of infants in a neonatal intensive care unit, children (and their parents) who could benefit from heart surgery, hospitalized children, diabetic adults, medical-surgical patients at risk for development of pressure ulcers, a spinal-cord injured patient, and hospice patients.

UNEXPECTED CHALLENGES AND OPPORTUNITIES

Although not totally unexpected, language and cultural differences proved to be more difficult than anticipated. For the Russians who spoke English and had Internet availability, project implementation and communication were enhanced. Otherwise, one of the conference coordinators who spends much of his time in Russia needed to serve as a go-between to facilitate communication. The distance and barriers to direct communication between the US and Russian collaborators created time lags in accomplishing our respective goals, at times leading to a loss of interest. These communication barriers also resulted in fewer opportunities for sharing of information and materials. This lessened the overall impact of collaborative opportunities. Distance and language barriers can easily make a project feel insurmountable. At times it was difficult for those involved to recapture the impetus of relating with a new colleague and the enthusiasm engendered by developing project goals while on the boat, especially if this was further complicated by language and time barriers. These projects were structured for a year's time with a report due at the end. The short timeframe was a benefit in that it created the need for momentum and an expectation which was fulfilled.

Another facet involving cultural differences is learning to judge the educational levels of the Russian nurses compared to their US colleagues to know how to share resources. At times it is easy to assume that if US and Russian nurses use the same words, they mean the same things. For example, the concept of *specialty* between the US and Russia is very different. Certainly the levels of educational preparation are very different, leading to differences in roles and responsibilities. Another obstacle encountered is the differences in nursing terminology and the structure of nursing practice. Even in the presence of a skilled interpreter, some nursing terms, such as primary nursing, even when translated exactly, are not understood because the concept does not exist in Russian nursing. This can often lead to misunderstanding between nurses. It's necessary to remember to avoid assumptions and to clarify information. Patience and a willingness to relearn are critical to successful and mutually successful working relationships.

LESSONS LEARNED

The effect that cultural differences can have on the planning process is a crucial factor in the success of the Conference Cruise. Therefore, working to understand the structure of Russian nursing, cultural biases, and how to address the language barrier are the most important tasks in the planning process; this actually sets the context for having constructive dialogue during the conference. Thus, two factors are essential to the success of this small grants program. One is a context that encourages dialogue to promote the connections necessary for collaborative relationships, and the second is a structure to support the funding and reporting to provide feedback about the completion of these projects.

WORDS OF WISDOM TO THOSE CONSIDERING INTERNATIONAL WORK

The projects resulting from the US-Russian Nursing Conference Cruise again demonstrate the power that networks and connections have in furthering collaboration, through which profound benefits are derived. In an editorial by Glass (2006), nurses are expanding nursing education opportunities to new places and spaces in response to the imperative for nursing to have a global perspective. This success story demonstrates both the intense interest of nurses to learn about challenges faced by nurses in other countries and to be helpful to each other. Additional contexts are needed to create opportunities for nurses to interact and dialogue for mutual learning about each other, about professional issues, and about cultural implications. Sharing a collaborative project provides the concrete basis for this mutual learning that is both enjoyable and effective. Through engaging in such collaborative networks and projects, nurses can meet a call for "nurses to embrace a global context … and contribute to the provision of health care that is based not on ethnocentrism but on an appreciation for differences among human beings and for an underlying common humanity across the globe and geographic boundaries" (Olshansky, 2006).

REFERENCES

Glass, N. (2006). Guest Editorial: Internationalizing nursing: Valuing the multiple places and spaces of nursing education. *Journal of Nursing Education*, 45(10): 387–388

Olshansky, E. (2006). Editorial: Nursing within a global context. *Journal of Professional Nursing*, 22(5): 263–264

8

Looking Back on 45 Years of International Nursing Involvement

Anne J. Davis, RN, PhD, DSc(hon), FAAN

The old adage "It is who you know and what you know" best describes my international nursing experience during the last 45 years because so much of it was the result of informal networks. Many invitations to lecture, teach courses, present at conferences, and work with graduate students occurred because of this network.

In 1962 I left my teaching position and personally funded two years living outside the United States (US). After visiting countries surrounding Israel, I spent a year living in Israel, where I taught for the Israeli Ministry of Health after working on a kibbutz and conducting a small study on negotiating privacy in a total institution. Then my network in psychiatry led me to a Danish mental hospital where I worked as a staff nurse in 1963 when I was not traveling about Europe. Over my 34 years at the University of California, San Francisco (UCSF), I met many international visitors and enrolled students who became friends, forming an important part of my large professional network. One of these visitors was the chief nurse of the Ministry of Health, Nigeria. When I was awarded a 1971 World Health Organization (WHO) Travel Fellowship to Ghana and Kenya, she obtained a short-term teaching position for me at the University of Ibadan, Nigeria, adding months to my stay in Africa. During the decade of the 1980s, I had a sabbatical in India, where I traveled extensively on my own funds learning about mental health problems. Later, invitations came to lecture in Spain, the United Kingdom (UK), Canada, Finland, Norway, Australia, New Zealand, Korea, and Colombia came.

Some of these invitations resulted from my writing a book with Mila Aroskar, *Ethical Dilemmas and Nursing Practice*, first published in 1978. The Citizen Ambassador Program invited me to take a group of nurses to The People's Republic of China in 1983. I was so impressed with Lin Ju Ying, president of the Chinese Nursing Association in Beijing, that I invited her to San Francisco. I raised funds from local institutions where Madam Lin spoke during her visit here. She and I became very close friends, and this relationship led to my annual lectures in China for about 20 years. Now I go annually to visit friends there.

When the journal *Nursing Ethics* began, the editor, Verena Tschudin, asked me to join and to help organize an international editorial board; my service continued for 10 years. Peer reviewing manuscripts from around the world provides insights into the nursing ethics world in special ways. Upon retirement from UCSF, a former doctoral student, Hiroko Minami, now International Council of Nurses (ICN) president, asked me to come to Japan to teach. This led to a new career at Nagano College of Nursing for six and a half years, where I taught all levels of nursing education and conducted research on issues in Japanese health-care ethics.

Returning home to San Francisco, two UK colleagues and I edited a book on teaching and learning nursing ethics (*Essentials of Teaching and Learning in Nursing Ethics: Perspectives and Methods*) written for an international audience and published in 2006. This year, 2007, I am working with doctoral (PhD) students on their research for two months at Hong Kong Polytechnic University and updating the Davis-Aroskar ethics book, now the Davis-Fowler book in its fifth edition. At the 2007 ICN meeting in Japan, I presented two papers reflecting my work with (1) women prisoners, human rights, and health in Australia, Canada, UK, and US and (2) activities of the International Nursing Ethics Center in the UK and its committee, Nurses for Human Rights and Health. I serve as the international president of this center.

FORMAL AND FORMAL-INFORMAL PROJECTS

While most of my international career has depended on informal networks, some aspects of it were more formal and went through organizations or were a mixture of formal and informal. Two research projects in China funded by the University of California Pacific Rim Research Fund examined problems experienced by chronically ill patients and their caregivers. A cross-cultural study, funded by the Institute of Nursing Research, focused on ethical problems in terminally ill Chinese-American, Hispanic-American, African-American, and Caucasian-American cancer patients and their families living in San Francisco. This study provided insights that helped me in international work.

My participation in two WHO projects focused on (1) female genital mutilation and (2) justice and informal care giving for chronically ill patients. This invitation came about because

Miriam Hirschfeld, WHO Chief Nurse Scientist, Geneva, had been a doctoral student at UCSF where I was her research advisor. So while the official invitation came from the WHO, my network facilitated the process.

In Japan Emiko Konishi and I obtained research monies annually from the Ministry of Education to examine aspects of nursing ethics, specifically the ethics of death and dying in that country. Emiko acted as a counterpart with me in this work.

A formal educational exchange program between Nagano College of Nursing and the National University of Samoa School of Nursing funded by Japan International Cooperation Association (JICA) grew from my informal visit to Samoa, where I took four undergraduate students with me to view Samoan nursing and to snorkel. I had the idea, but it was Dean Takako Mitoh who obtained funding for this ongoing exchange program.

On my second working visit to Korea, colleagues suggested that I apply to the Fulbright Senior Specialist Project and return to Yonsei University to work with PhD students and give lectures on nursing ethics. The UCSF nursing school dean sent out e-mail saying that Kaohsiung Medical University, Taiwan, was interested in inviting someone to teach for one month. So, I said if they were interested in ethics, I could go, and I did so. This was funded by the university there, as other such invitations to universities in many countries had been. My philosophy is to provide in-kind support for developing countries and to seek funding from those that are already developed. Money gleaned from the developed countries helps to defray costs incurred during my in-kind work.

SELECTED OUTCOMES ACHIEVED

Many outcomes have resulted from my long and rich international career that include the following:

1. Raising important health-related and ethical questions about health-care practice in general and nursing practice specifically. There are many examples in several countries.

2. Publishing research findings used by colleagues. For example, Dr. Thomas Lambo, WHO, Geneva, used my article on native healers. Nurses internationally read my publications, and some contact me.

3. Having an impact on students and colleagues especially in Japan. For example, I remain connected to former students and colleagues there who ask for help and advice.

4. Acting as midwife to connect people with similar interests, for example, the Good Nurse Research Project being conducted in Japan, China, Hong Kong, Taiwan, and Korea.

5. Starting the Nagano College of Nursing–National University of Samoa educational exchange program still being funded by Joint Commission International (JCI).

CHALLENGES AND OPPORTUNITIES

Many times what might be defined as a challenge is actually an opportunity. I never felt alone in my work, but always thought I could ask and receive the help I needed in understanding and coping with a situation. Funding is available, so write a good proposal and apply.

LESSONS LEARNED

So many lessons have been learned, and some are now such an integral part of me that it is difficult to remember that I learned them in international work:

1. You can only be yourself, but that self should be as informed as possible about the culture in which you are working. Read everything you possibly can including novels, poetry, history, social science studies, health reports, and nursing journals.

2. Communicate in ways that others, whose first language is not English, can understand.

3. Understand that people are busy with complex lives, so find ways to work alone at times and entertain yourself. Colleagues are usually hospitable, but they have many obligations to attend to also.

4. Rather than saying something like, "In the US, we do it this way," ask a question for clarification. Be open to other ways of thinking and doing.

5. In part, you are always dependant on others for understanding the world at hand and also in practical ways. Accept help gracefully.

6. Be careful what you say no to.

7. I think that the concept of cultural competency is misguided and possibly leads to problems. Be culturally sensitive and know you are ignorant. You will learn just how ignorant you really are as time goes along.

WORDS OF ADVICE

1. Be sure that you can be alone.

2. Be careful that you do not become a person without a country. It might be better for some people, like me, to have a home base and work internationally but not in a full-time career.

3. Be open to new experiences and friendly to people.

4. Eat almost anything. Travel on almost anything. Do not be fussy about daily life aspects. One reason you are there is that it is different from home.

5. Make friendships that last, which means working to keep them going.

6. Know your strengths and limitations and act accordingly.

7. Have fun, but don't often tell jokes because they are usually culturally embedded and limited.

8. Read as much as possible before you go and talk with anyone who has been there.

9. Work with another person in a counterpart role whether assigned or not.

10. Put back into the common pot and help others who want to work internationally.

CONCLUSION

Nursing displays a remarkable camaraderie that I do not see in the same way in other professional groups. This helpful attitude can also be found in some other travelers. People ask me how I can go off around the world, and I answer, because someone always helps me if I need it. In Ethiopia, the hospital matron invited me to stay in her home when I could not find a hotel room because of the conference in town. And other people also give aid. In Hyderabad, India, when I became ill and fainted, the lamp shade salesman from Madras was not only most helpful that evening, but also stopped by next morning to check on me before he left to go home. One of the most important items you will need in international work is trust of others. You may be disappointed, but not often. And you will need to be trusted by others as well, which means that you need to think about your behavior and how it might be perceived by those others. In the final analysis, it is who you know and what you know and how you act that make for a rich, rewarding, and fruitful international career in nursing. I know that for a fact. More than 45 years of international nursing has enriched me personally and professionally; I, in turn, have enriched the lives of others.

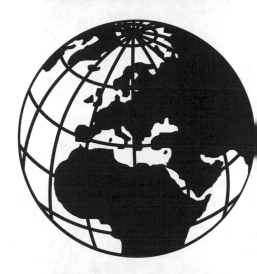

NUMBERS

B

C

I

M

N

O–P